The Happiness Diet

The Happiness Diet

A Nutritional Prescription for
a Sharp Brain, Balanced Mood,
and Lean, Energized Body

Tʏʟᴇʀ Gʀᴀʜᴀᴍ ᴀɴᴅ Dʀᴇᴡ Rᴀᴍsᴇʏ, **MD**

RODALE.

© 2011 by Tyler Graham and Drew Ramsey, MD

All rights reserved. No part of this publication may be reproduced or transmitted in any form or by any means, electronic or mechanical, including photocopying, recording, or any other information storage and retrieval system, without the written permission of the publisher.

Rodale books may be purchased for business or promotional use or for special sales. For information, please write to:

Special Markets Department, Rodale, Inc., 733 Third Avenue, New York, NY 10017

Printed in the United States of America

Rodale Inc. makes every effort to use acid-free ♾, recycled paper ♺.

Book design by Christina Gaugler

Library of Congress Cataloging-in-Publication Data is on file with the publisher.

ISBN 978-1-60529-327-1

Distributed to the trade by Macmillan

2 4 6 8 10 9 7 5 3 1   hardcover

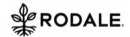

We inspire and enable people to improve their lives and the world around them.

www.rodalebooks.com

This book is dedicated to America's farmers.

Contents

Acknowledgments

First we'd like to thank Rodale for all the support they've given to this project. We especially appreciate Julie Will's and Karen Rinaldi's votes of confidence in us in the middle of a recession. We'd also like to thank Gena Smith and Zachary Greenwald for their many late nights, as well as Colin Dickerman and Pam Krauss for helping us to the finish line. Emily Weber and Yelena Nesbit, we appreciate your wise counsel. Heather Jackson, you are a book publishing sage. Joy Tutela, you are a patient, patient woman. Thank you so much for going above and beyond.

Tyler would like to start by thanking his mother, who made sure that most nights the Graham family sat down together for a home-cooked meal. He'd also like to thank his father for making a wholesome breakfast each morning. A big, warm thanks to those who have long supported Tyler (John and Isabel Joynt, John Graham, Juli, Kris, Dana, Dickie Lee) and to those who will in the future (Carter, Sterling, Colton, Lexi, Brynlee). A special thanks to the special team at *Best Life*. This book would not have been possible without friends like Bone and Karen, Jason Adams, Josh Dean, Colin O'Banion, Jeff Surowka, Jenny, and Joel Weber. Nor would it have been possible without the wisdom of some very special counsel for SRL, such as John Casalena, Gordon Zuckerman, and Rick Hamilton. Thanks to the smart, thoughtful minds of people like Michael Pollan, Gary Taubes, and Marion Nestle whose writings make our country a better place in which to live and to eat. And a very special thanks to Miss Mieke ten Have.

Drew thanks his parents for taking a leap and returning to the land and his patients, who teach him about the power of food and challenge him to be a better physician daily. He graciously thanks Columbia University's Department of Psychiatry and the New York State Psychiatric Institute, where he has been privileged to train and now to teach. The faculty's tireless pursuit of a better understanding of the brain and better treatments has been a constant inspiration. Special thanks to his colleagues who read early drafts and provided wise counsel, particularly Phil Muskin, Dan Chrzanowski, and David Schab, and also to Marcia Lux, Julian Abrams, and Lars Lund who have continued to make him a better doctor ever since intern year. Bob Wise has served as an invaluable mentor and provided detailed comments and exceptional counsel. MVA would be proud. Additionally, the guidance of Ron Rieder, Pel Sarti, and Ron Puddu has made this book possible. Drew thanks his dear friends for their unwavering support and his wife Lucy for being the ideal partner in life and in parenting: patient, thoughtful, and firm about the need for food and sleep. He thanks Greta for making life's priorities clear.

Introduction

What if you discovered that the best place to begin your personal pursuit of happiness is at the end of your fork? Emerging research from the fields of neuroscience and nutrition shows that by changing what you eat, you can improve your mental and emotional well-being. You can stabilize your moods. You can improve your focus. You can even make your brain grow.

So what do we mean by happiness? There have been many books published in recent years that explore different approaches to attaining happiness—some from motivational speakers, others from experts in the field of positive psychology. At their core these are suggestions for behavioral changes that are meant to improve your psychological well-being and outlook on life. We are coming at this from a very different perspective: Before you start changing your outlook on life to improve your emotional well-being, we want to make sure your eating behavior is the best it can be so that the master mood regulator—the brain—is provided with what it needs to be strong, sharp, healthy . . . and happy.

Increasingly, in our experience, it seems that fewer people truly feel they have control over their diet. "It's just too hard to eat right," we often hear. "Everyone says something different" is another refrain we get a lot. We want to change this state of affairs and settle the confusion about what needs to be eaten for a happy, healthy brain and body. The Happiness Diet provides concrete tools (tasty ones, too) for doing just that.

But as modern Americans, we face some formidable and largely invisible obstacles in seeking happiness. The food we eat each day is undermining our emotional and mental well-being. Many of the nutrients that human brains depend on for healthy functioning have been stripped from our food supply by factory farming and by modern methods of food processing. Compounding these losses, new chemicals have been added that impair our brain functioning. You're probably well aware that our food is responsible for our epidemic levels of obesity and diabetes, but you might be surprised that it's also largely responsible for skyrocketing levels of brain disorders. We all want to be happy, but every day most of us consume what amounts to a series of "Unhappy Meals."

Thanks to the introduction of industrial-scale food processing, Americans have changed their dietary habits more in the past 100 years than all of humanity had in the previous 100,000. The Modern American Diet—we call it the MAD—is characterized first and foremost by simple sugars and refined carbohydrates now found in everything from cereal to pasta. These sugars play tricks on your brain, so you keep craving more and more of them, even though sugar consumption actually contributes to the *shrinkage* of key areas of your brain responsible for everything from memories to mood regulation.

The second largest source of calories in the MAD are added fats—refined vegetable and seed oils that have high amounts of omega-6 fats as well as trans fats, which have been linked to an increased risk of depression. A third critical aspect of the MAD most detrimental to our brain functions is the factory farming of cows, pigs, chickens, and even fish. Not only are these creatures pumped full of antibiotics and hormones to promote their growth, but they feed on an unnatural diet of grain, which leaves their flesh deficient in many of the very fats and nutrients our brains have required from animals since the dawn of humankind. Strange as it seems, with the MAD you can expand your waistline and starve your brain at the same time, which is exactly what growing numbers of Americans are doing.

Study after study in the medical research journals confirm that people who are most dependent on MAD-style eating habits have increased levels of depression, anxiety, mood swings, hyperactivity, and a wide variety of other mental and emotional problems. Our belief, backed up by ample research, is that the best way to prevent the MAD assault on our health and happiness is to go back to eating the wholesome foods that nurtured the development of our brains over tens of thousands of years of evolution.

Let's take a closer look at the cheeseburger on the cover of the book. To many nutritionists, this is a snapshot of everything that is wrong with the American diet: It's fatty, full of cholesterol, and high in calories. In the Happiness Diet, though, our burger is an important source for much of what you and your brain need for healthy growth and high functioning. The reason is that this is not your typical fast-food burger. The cheese and meat both came from grass-fed cows, ensuring you will get a good supply of brain-healthy omega-3s and other nutrients not found in factory-farmed animals. The lettuce and tomatoes were organically grown, so they offer the maximum number of valuable nutrients such as folate and lycopene without the risks of pesticides. The bun is made of whole grains, so it includes magnesium, zinc, B vitamins, and fiber instead of the empty calories in your typical bun.

· · · · · · · · ·

So, aside from the occasional burger, what can you expect from the Happiness Diet?

In Part 1, we define what we mean by happiness. We believe that you can't work toward this desirable state of mind if your brain's machinery isn't well oiled and firing on all cylinders. We go on a short tour of the nutrients needed for a healthy brain to work and why food choice plays such an important role in either optimizing or diminishing its functions. Our next stop is a look at how our food has changed—how a few wrong turns down the nutrition highway wrecked our health and happiness.

This brief history lesson is key to understanding how so many unhappy meals have come into our food supply.

We next walk you through the hall of shame: the most common culprits that are collectively destroying our mood. The sugar, fats, toxins, and pesticides in the MAD make up a modern chemistry lab concoction that is lacking the key ingredients for a healthy brain. We go into all the details of how sugar assaults the brain so effectively that it's our number one mood buster. We explain why processed foods full of additives and preservatives are also bad for your brain. We'll see how researchers are showing a clearer link between obesity and depression, and why some are so convinced of the dietary component to Alzheimer's disease that they have nicknamed it "type 3" diabetes.

Once we move beyond what we're doing wrong with our MAD choices, we share the Essential Elements that will later form the core of the Happiness Diet. These are the best foods from which to get these vitamins, minerals, and other phytonutrients: healthier sugars (yes, there is such a thing), meat, fats, milk, eggs, and a huge array of plants. We've studied hundreds of books and medical journals, so we're as up-to-date as possible in the fast-changing world of nutrition science. Our research leads us to some surprising recommendations for health foods and mood boosters, including beef, bacon, and eggs, and explains what you need to do to best keep your brain well-fed.

In Part 2, we share what science knows about what we call "focus foods." In "Food for Thought," we suggest you amp up the intake of these specific nutrients and foods to enhance brain function, cognition, and sharpness. The chapter that follows, "Food for Energy," shows you what to eat to maximize energy levels, so you're soon fully recharged. With "Food for Good Mood," you'll find out about the best choices for taming tension and anxiety while stabilizing and boosting mood.

After we've covered what to eat, we'll show you where to shop and how to stock your kitchen. Our two-week menu plan, which includes some of our own personal favorite recipes, should assure you that you don't need to be a culinary expert to prepare and enjoy delicious brain-healthy meals. Eating the right foods to best enhance brain function should be part of everyone's goal at every meal. Feel free to mix and match the menus; they're all good for you and for your state of mind.

Don't get us wrong: We don't believe in magic bullets. We do believe in good science and the cumulative effects of eating the broad array of these "happy" foods each and every day. The whole is definitely greater than the sum of its parts when it comes to any diet, including ours. No one food is going to be the superstar of this plan, but there are super-foods (those rich in the Essential Elements of Happiness), and we're going to give you a slew of the best ones to choose from for optimal mental health.

We can take control of what we eat, but it's not going to always be easy. You didn't get to a place of making the wrong food choices without a lot of pushing from the food industry and marketers from Madison Avenue. That is why throughout the book we provide some needed background on how we came to be eating in a way that's so destructive for our collective mental health. Peppered throughout, you will find this information in sidebars and in the margins. We've included a running list of 100 good reasons to avoid processed food (just look at number 23 and the ingredients list for this Oscar Meyer Lunchable and you'll never pack it in your kids' lunch again). We also provide brief history lessons on how so many unhappy meals have come into our food supply. Knowing this background acts as just another layer of motivation—and protection—as you change your course and get on a happier, smoother path.

If you need any further incentive, consider this: Another bonus that comes from following this diet is serious weight loss. It's almost impossible *not* to lose weight once you step off the MAD merry-go-round of sugar crashes and cravings. And you'll discover some pretty controversial, maybe even shocking, information about mood and obesity, too.

We hope that through this book, you will grasp just how important food is to your short-term mental and emotional state and your long-term moods and mental functions. We want you to feel that you are able to change not only your body but your brain as well.

Stick with us, and you'll feel great. Period.

Eat this way for life and you'll find that you're engaging with the world in a way that spreads this happiness to others.

Why not try it?

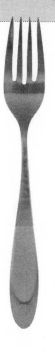

Part 1

This Is Your Brain
ON FOOD

1

What Is Happiness?

We take for granted that the brain is the seat of human consciousness, but it's been less than 200 years since scientists even began to understand how the brain functions. The ancient Egyptians thought so little of the brain that they discarded the gray matter inside the skull like a piece of trash during the process of mummification, while setting aside and preserving the valuable heart, lungs, and intestines for use in the afterlife.

Greek philosophers debated the brain's importance, and Aristotle deemed it an organ "of minor importance," speculating that it acted as a radiator to keep the body from overheating. Hippocrates, the father of modern medicine, saw things differently: "Man ought to know that from nothing else but the brain come the joys, delight, laughter, sports and sorrows, griefs, despondency, and lamentations." Obviously, we now agree with him. He's also famous for another aphorism that we're especially fond of: "Let thy food be thy medicine and let thy medicine be thy food."

The first detailed anatomical atlas of the brain, *Cerebri Anatome*, was published in 1664 by Thomas Willis. And the notion that electrical currents flow through human tissue, a basic property of the nervous system, was first described a little over two hundred years ago by Luigi Galvani, who observed "animal electricity" flowing through the body. But it wasn't until the 1800s and the invention of new tissue-staining techniques, coupled with the compound microscope, that scientists could actually see the basic building blocks of the brain. Heinrich Wilhelm Gottfried von Waldeyer-Hartz, a German anatomist, named these cells "neurons" in 1891. Only very recently have new imaging technologies, like functional magnetic resonance imaging (fMRI) and positron-emission tomography (PET), allowed scientists to observe neurons in action. After thousands of years of speculating on the nature of the brain, we are only now beginning to unravel how it works.

This Is Your Brain

The human brain is a three-pound wrinkly, gray organ that sits suspended in a fluid cushion inside the skull. While the brain accounts for about 2 percent of your body's weight, it burns 20 percent of your body's fuel. That's because the brain is the body's command center—the most complex supercomputer ever created. It's constantly processing unfathomable amounts of information. While you are running errands around town, for example, your brain is keeping track and regulating your heart rate, blood sugar, temperature, the pressure applied to the gas pedal, the sounds inside and outside the car, the speed of each automobile within vision, and an unconscious memory of nearly every image that passes by at a speed of sixty miles per hour.

We've all heard the old adage that we don't use 90 percent of our brains, but the reality is that we're consciously aware of only about 10 percent of what our brain is doing. The brain has more than one hundred billion neurons. Each one of these cells can be connected by synapses to ten thousand other neurons. Harvard psychiatrist John Ratey, MD, estimates that, mathematically speaking, the number of electrochemical con-

figurations possible in the brain is on the order of ten to the trillionth
power. This means there are more connections in a single human brain
then there are cubic feet in the universe.

These billions of neurons don't directly connect to one another, but
are separated by junctions known as synapses. Messages travel from neuron to neuron with the aid of brain chemicals called neurotransmitters.
Once enough neurotransmitter builds up in the synapse, the brain cell
fires and tells other brain cells to fire, creating a ripple effect. This communication is what happens when we figure out a crossword puzzle
answer, laugh at joke, or cry about something sad.

Some neurotransmitters, such as serotonin, adrenaline, and dopamine, have become household names, well-known for the their abilities to
affect mood and behavior. Promoting the release of dopamine is how the
caffeine in your morning coffee gets your day started. But there are hundreds of others, and, depending on the receptor it touches, a neurotransmitter like serotonin can trigger either the constriction or relaxation of
blood vessels, nausea or hunger, an orgasm or the loss of libido. This complex biological machinery is also what ultimately determines how we feel.
It's also, of course, made out of the food you eat.

This Is Your Brain on Food

As the Modern American Diet has changed in the past 100 years, so have
our brains. That's partly because the MAD diet has replaced many mood-
boosting animal fats like docosahexaenoic acid (DHA) and conjugated

TOP 100 REASONS TO AVOID PROCESSED FOODS

The greater the number of cheap cuts of meat ground into a single patty, the greater the risk of contamination with *E. coli*. A standard fast-food hamburger contains the trimmings of dozens of cows raised around the globe.

linoleic acid (CLA) with new vegetable fats derived largely from corn and soy that humans rarely ever consumed before. MAD foods are also devoid of many vitamins, minerals, and phytonutrient compounds found in plants that were once staples of the American dinner table. Instead, we're eating new foods grown and harvested in factories. And to create palatable, presentable products to the public, food processors add artificial dyes (linked to many brain disorders), preservatives (linked to cancer and weight gain), and synthetic nutrients (linked to cancer, asthma, and infertility).

If you eat a diet missing any of the essential elements needed by your brain to function, what seems a minor imbalance can have a major effect. Our brains have co-evolved with certain varieties of foods over thousands of years. From our brains to those of our most distant ancestors, there is a continuous genetic chain of nutrition that has been broken by MAD substitutions, innovations, and prohibitions, none of which have stood the test of time in the same way as grass-fed beef, free-range eggs, and organic vegetables and fruits. This book wants to reforge that link to a tradition of eating that has always produced healthy, happy people whenever good food has been in abundance.

Consider what might happen to you if you are running low on iron, a condition shared by about 15 percent of American women of reproductive age. Inadequate stores of iron diminish your body's ability to transport oxygen in the blood. Several molecules needed for the proper connections to occur between your brain cells, such as the neurotransmitters dopamine and serotonin, require iron for their synthesis.

You start the day in your iron-deficient state, coaxed out of bed by a loud alarm. Your limbs feel heavy. Your head feels groggy, like the morning after you've had one too many drinks. Your wake-up routine is tough: you misplaced your keys, you feel rushed, and the short walk to work gets you winded. You go to the gym, but then you get light-headed on the treadmill. You tend to lose patience more easily. You get frustrated with your kids and you snap at your spouse. Over a few weeks the combination of fatigue, bad mood, and lack of concentration starts to fray your life. A ripple of unhappiness begins to spread, and it all began with a set of choices made at mealtimes over the past few months.

Wherever the MAD diet goes, rates of depression tend to rise. The disease has become the leading cause of disability in middle- and high-income countries around the world. A large study recently published in the *British Journal of Psychiatry* found that eating processed foods, such as refined carbohydrates, sweets, and processed meats, increased the risk of depression by about 60 percent. Eating a whole-food diet, on the other hand, decreased the risk of depression by about 26 percent.

The most common medical treatments for depression, of course, are medication and psychotherapy—not diet. Although both have been remarkably effective for many people, it makes sense to use a diversity of strategies when it comes to caring for our brains. On a societal level, these problems with diet and brain function may seem insurmountable, though we hold out hope that change over time is possible. On an individual level, however, we've found that overcoming the MAD's ill effects with the Happiness Diet can be quite simple and immediate.

TOP 100 REASONS TO AVOID PROCESSED FOODS

3

A Dunkin' Donuts glazed chocolate cake stick contains more than forty ingredients, including five different types of gums and TBHQ, a form of butane (lighter fluid) that's used as a preservative.

Your Mind Is Your Body

There is no separation between the mind and the body. A sickened body almost always impairs the mind. A handful of new studies show that people who are diabetic, obese, or suffering from cardiovascular disease perform worse on cognitive tests than those who are leaner and healthier. New research from Kent State University in Ohio showed that obese patients who received weight reduction surgery improved their cognitive functioning within a few weeks. In other words, the mere fact of being obese impairs the wiring of the human brain.

Everywhere we hear how rates of obesity and adult-onset diabetes are soaring. Rates of obesity and depression have both doubled in recent decades, and they are deeply interconnected epidemics. Today two out of three Americans are overweight and one in four over the age of twenty has something known as prediabetes, an impaired ability to regulate blood sugar that speeds up the process of aging. That's seventy-nine million adults.

Both obesity and diabetes wreak havoc on brain health. Patients with diabetes have much higher rates of depression, as do those who have other diseases associated with obesity such as heart disease and cancer. As people with these diseases age, their brains have been shown to shrink. Thanks to the imaging techniques mentioned earlier, we know that specific areas linked to positive emotions and clear thinking, like the hippocampus and hypothalamus, are specifically at risk. Studies show that the brains of the obese appear sixteen years older than those of people of normal weight.

TOP 100 REASONS TO AVOID PROCESSED FOODS

Eating a diet high in fast food appears to cause an abnormal buildup of tau protein tangles in the brain—similar to what happens in those diagnosed with Alzheimer's disease.

The larger the belly size, the larger your risk of dementia and depression.

Here is just a sampling of some important recent studies attesting to the importance of food to your happiness and well-being. In the back of this book you will see documentation for many more.

- A study of 54,632 women by the Harvard School of Public Health found that those who ate the *most* omega-3s and the *least* omega-6s were significantly less likely to suffer from depression.
- Research involving 12,059 college graduates over an average of 6.6 years found that the more trans fats participants ate, the *more likely* they were to be depressed. Those who ate the most trans fats had a 48 percent increased risk.
- When the dietary habits of 4,856 people were followed for more than ten years, researchers found that the women who consumed the most oleic acid, the predominant fat in olive oil and lard, were the *least likely* to report a severe depressed mood. The men who ate the most linoleic acid, the main fat in soybean and corn oils, were found to be *most likely* to get depressed.
- A six-week experiment involving children with attention deficit/ hyperactivity disorder revealed that a diet restricted to simple whole foods like meat, rice, vegetables, pears, and water resulted in significant behavioral improvement for 78 percent of the children. Once they were placed back on a MAD, 63 percent suffered worse ADHD symptoms.
- A test of the cognitive functions of 280 healthy middle-aged community volunteers discovered that those with the highest blood levels of the omega-3 fatty acid DHA performed significantly better on tests of nonverbal reasoning, working memory, and vocabulary.

Some of these studies show more conclusive results than others, but the one result you will never see is one that shows that the MAD improves

5

TOP 100 REASONS TO AVOID PROCESSED FOODS

It takes no time to decode the list of ingredients on an apple—there isn't one.

cognitive function. Or that MAD foods deter depression. Or that those whose diets rely on MAD sugars and vegetable oils have lower rates of anxiety, dementia, or depression. The MAD is a hands-down loser when it comes to your mental, emotional, and physical well-being. It is so bad for you that you must wonder how such a thing could ever develop and what the people who created it were thinking. Here's a hint: They weren't always thinking about your happiness.

A Three-Point Plan for Happiness

To best explain how your food affects how you feel, we're going to separate your "happiness ability" into three areas of brain function. The first area is **cognitive functioning,** which is your overall capacity to focus, think, plan, and remember. Lost your keys? Can't remember a colleague's name? Where *did* you park that car? Getting stuck at work on complex problems? While we all experience some decline in these abilities as we age, studies have pointed to beneficial effects from Happiness Diet essential elements such as omega-3s, tocotrienols, vitamins B_{12} and B_6, and folates, which are all abundant in whole foods. (If you think you can match the power of whole foods with supplements, see page 222.)

The second area of brain function that food affects is **emotional regulation.** Overreacting, temper on high, motor constantly humming . . . all are signs that your brain is dysregulated and that your emotions aren't fully under your control. If your lows and highs are balanced, your overall mood will be more even and your reactions will be much more in check. It's the difference between blowing up in traffic or not, yelling at

YOUR EVER-EXPANDING PLASTIC BRAIN

What if we told you that there's a molecule that could make your brain grow? What sounds like a pitch for a new supplement is actually a molecule at the frontier of modern neuroscience. The twentieth century ended with a scientific discovery that rocked the world: Your brain is not fixed—it can expand, get smarter, and make virtually everything in life easier to deal with. It's all due to a special protein called brain-derived neurotrophic factor (BDNF) that's been called by many scientists as Miracle-Gro for the brain. More BDNF means you've got a brain primed for learning, good moods, and clear thinking. Reduce BDNF levels in the brain and you feel blue, forget things, and can't learn. Increase BDNF and brain areas central to thinking and feeling look healthy and robust, with their neurons making thousands of connections. The effective treatment of clinical depression is associated with increased BDNF levels. You can increase the BDNF level in your brain simply by changing the foods you eat. Eat more processed, high-sugar foods and BDNF levels go down. Eat foods with plenty of folate, vitamin B$_{12}$, or omega-3 and your BDNF levels go up. Keep reading and you'll be well on your way.

your kids or talking to them, being devastated that a new love hasn't phoned or diving into a great new book. Research into depression, in particular, has shown that processed foods high in sugar, omega-6 fats, and trans fats are all associated with higher rates of depression, while consumption of oleic acid, omega-3s, and whole foods such as fish, meats, fruits, and vegetables was associated with lowered rates of depression.

Anxiety is third area of brain function affected by food. Anxiety is endemic in the modern world—too many e-mails to return, bills to pay, school applications to complete. There has never before been as much to worry about, but anxiety is a tricky emotion. It can be a great motivator.

TOP 100 REASONS TO AVOID PROCESSED FOODS

6

According to a study from researchers at UCLA, it takes only *two months* to lower levels of brain chemicals responsible for learning and memory (like BDNF) on a steady diet of processed foods.

We often perform our greatest feats under tremendous stress: It provides the "juice" to power us through a stressful meeting or the focus needed to finish an important report. For that reason, it's important to protect our brains from the noise of needless worry. This anxiety disrupts both cognitive functioning and emotional regulation; with excess worry, you don't think clearly and instead spin your wheels. Again, studies have shown

FLYING RIGHT: THE HD GUIDE TO NEUROTRANSMITTERS

While we hear a lot about the so-called happiness molecule serotonin, we know today that mood and brain function depend on dozens and dozens of neurotransmitters. Below are just a few of the brain's neurotransmitters and the foods you use to make them; this list will give you a hint of just how complex the command center of your body—and your life—really is.

GLUTAMATE
What it does: Glutamate is the most common neurotransmitter in the brain. It promotes the firing of other neurons and is involved in learning, cognition, and regulating the formation of new brain cells.
How to make it: Whole wheat toast and eggs.

GLYCINE
What it does: Glycine makes neurons less likely to fire and regulates vision and movement. By influencing the growth of new neuron connections (synaptic plasticity), it works in concert with glutamate to stimulate certain receptors in the brain (NMDA) that underlie learning and memory.
How to make it: Pork chops with a side of sautéed spinach, topped with sesame seeds.

GABA
What it does: GABA is the second most common neurotransmitter in the brain. It balances glutamate by making neurons less likely to fire. The calming effects of alcohol and sedatives like Valium and Xanax are caused by their stimulating of GABA receptors.
How to make it: Flank steak and mashed potatoes with garlic, leeks, or shallots.

SEROTONIN
What it does: Serotonin is a major regulator of mood, appetite, sex drive, pain, sleep/wake cycle, alertness, body temperature, blood clotting, and

evidence that the Modern American Diet of refined carbohydrates and sugary treats contributes to excess anxiety. One study of middle-aged and elderly adults found the highest rates of anxiety disorders among those whose blood showed low levels of the nutrient choline, which is found abundantly in eggs and fish. A malnourished brain creates a worried mind.

The pursuit of happiness takes consistent effort. This is why a lean,

digestion. Markers of low serotonin in the brain are linked with low mood, aggression, irritability, and suicide.
How to make it: Oven-roasted cod, a side of clams, and fruit salad.

NOREPINEPHRINE
What it does: Norepinephrine is involved in learning, focus, mood, the formation of new brain cells, decreasing brain inflammation, regulating blood pressure, and our flight-or-fight response. It is also the neurotransmitter most affected by Alzheimer's disease.
How to make it: Roasted chicken with red potatoes and blue cheese.

DOPAMINE
What it does: Dopamine helps regulate pleasure, energy, mood, learning, focus, sleep, and memory. It is believed that obese people get less pleasure from food because they have fewer dopamine receptors, which is one theory why they may eat more. Stimulants like nicotine, caffeine, amphetamines, and cocaine all increase dopamine release. Patients with Parkinson's disease are slowed down because of a lack of dopamine.
How to make it: Scrambled eggs with a side of dark, leafy greens.

ANANDAMIDE
What it does: Anandamide binds to our brains' cannabinoid receptors (those also affected by marijuana) and regulates memory, mood, hunger, pleasure, and the growth of new brain cells. Unlike most other neurotransmitters, which are made from amino acids, anandamide is made from fat. The name is derived from the Sanskrit word for bliss.
How to make it: Salmon with kale sautéed in olive oil and topped with goat cheese.

TOP 100 REASONS TO AVOID PROCESSED FOODS

Twenty-eight different pesticide residues have been identified in mass-produced applesauce, including carbaryl, a neurotoxin, and carbendazim, a hormone disruptor.

energized body is so vital to cognitive functioning, emotional regulation, and anxiety. When you have a lot of energy, cognitive tasks feel easier to accomplish, frustrations are easier to bear, and anxiety is less likely to overwhelm you. With proper brain nutrition, you create a strong foundation from which you can create the life you want. Here's our formula for brain happiness in its simplest, three-point form.

- Clear thinking and focused attention = a greater ability to plan and execute.
- Steady and content moods = a greater ability to absorb the frustrations of life and regulate your emotions.
- Freedom from needless worry = turning your wheels, not spinning them.
  PLUS
- Energy to engage = a vibrant pursuit of all of life's possibilities.

Achieving these ideals is possible only through a well-fed, well-nourished brain. It is interesting, though, that nearly all the most common prescriptions for improving cognitive functioning involve mental exercises such as puzzle-solving, and most treatments for emotional regulation and anxiety lean toward psychotherapy and medication. These remedies all have their benefits, but dietary change is rarely suggested as a partial remedy— even though the brain, like any other body organ, is highly reliant on a good diet for proper functioning. That's why we've created the Happiness Diet. But before we get to all the solutions, we want to take you on a quick spin through how we all get misled in the hope that it'll help keep you mindful of your dietary changes. It won't be too difficult, we promise.

2

A Brief History of the Modern American Diet

A lot has changed in the last few hundred years that has led us to our MAD way of life, and it's our hope that a quick tour through these changes will help you understand why being mindful of what you eat is so important to staying healthy and happy. If you stick with us here, we promise you'll gain a much greater understanding of why simple dietary changes can have such drastic impacts on your health.

For most of humanity's existence, no one worried about overeating. No one worried about consuming too much fat or not eating enough antioxidants. In a world without refrigerators and freezers, one of the most important concerns was keeping food fresh.

When food wasn't fresh, it was often doctored with spice, which is why, at one time, the exports of the Spice Islands in the Indian Ocean were more valuable than silver or gold. The extraordinary value of spices prompted Christopher Columbus to sail west to find a new route to the East and prove that the world was round. When he arrived on the island of Hispaniola, he described the spicy native chili fruits as "pepper" because that's what he was looking for. That's why we call jalapeños and habaneros "chile *peppers*" rather than simply "chiles"—as they'd been known for thousands of years. While Columbus hadn't in fact discovered the Spice Islands, his discovery of North America did usher in the biggest exchange of food and food-producing technologies in the history of humanity.

When Columbus returned to Spain, he also brought back something else to the European continent: corn. Native Americans cultivated hundreds of varieties of corn: red, blue; some the width of a finger, others as wide as a child's forearm; some bitter, some sweet. They soaked it overnight with the mineral lime and then ground the corn into a paste and cooked it into tortillas. Corn soon became a peasant staple across Europe: It was eaten as a thick porridge in England; Italians called it polenta, Romanians called it mămăligă, and Hungarians called it puliszka. (Southerners in the United States later developed their own version: grits.) The only problem with this widespread adoption of corn was that the Europeans neglected the important step of presoaking the corn in slack lime, a process known today as nixtamalization. This process releases vitamin B_3, also known as niacin.

By the 1700s, strange reports of a ghastly new species of humans were emerging from Eastern Europe. These creatures were sensitive to light and rarely ventured out during the day. Their skin was extremely pale and often flaked off at the touch. They were very anxious, often attacked bystanders, and were notorious for eating all manner of strange foods such as spiders and flies. But nothing was stranger than their reputed thirst for human blood. Their bloodstained teeth and gums were

TOP 100 REASONS TO AVOID PROCESSED FOODS

Processed food is only as good as its packaging: In the summer of 2010, Kellogg's recalled twenty-eight million boxes of cereal because a compound in the box lining (they wouldn't say what) was giving off a foul smell and tainting the taste of the boxed foods.

TOP 100 REASONS TO AVOID PROCESSED FOODS

According to the National Toxicology Program, butylated
hydroxyanisole (BHA), a preservative used in McDonald's sausage,
among other foods, is suspected to be a human carcinogen.

proof of this. And it was said that if you came into close contact with one
of these tortured souls, you, too, might become one yourself: a vampire.
How's that for bad mood food?

Today, we call this disease by another name, pellagra. It comes from
a deficiency of the essential vitamin B$_3$, caused in this case when the European peasantry switched from other grains to corn without keeping the
traditional preparation of adding lime. Without vitamin B$_3$, our nervous
system deteriorates, we become agitated, our eyes become extremely sensitive to light, our skin becomes pale and brittle, we develop open sores
around the mouth, and we get aggressive. We turn into vampires.

Pellagra may be an extreme example, but as humans adopted new
foods and abandoned traditional sources, nutrional deficiencies that cause
severe problems with mental functioning became common. Prior to 1900,
in West Virginia there had never been a case of goiter, "a food-deficiency
disease which causes feeble-mindedness, deaf-mutism, and general physical and mental degeneration from one generation to the next." But in the
early twentieth century, West Virginians swapped the local coarse,
brownish salt from the Kanawha River for the "refined and free flowing"
salt from Michigan and Ohio, and soon goiter become endemic in the
state. A survey of schoolgirls in 1922 found that 60 percent suffered from
the disorder. The imported salt from what became known as the "goiter
belt" lacked iodine, a nutrient essential for proper brain development.

· · · · · · · · ·

The study of illnesses caused by nutritional deficiency led to the discovery
of vitamins. It's a word that was coined in 1911 by Casimir Funk, who com-

TOP 100 REASONS TO AVOID PROCESSED FOODS

The same company that makes metal detectors for airports also sells them to food manufacturers, who use the devices to test processed meats for stray wires, metal shards, and hypodermic needles.

bined the words *vital* and *amine* to describe the substance he isolated from the husk of rice. It had been reported that the husk contained a substance that prevented beriberi, a medical condition characterized by severe lethargy, confusion, emotional problems, and heart failure. Funk had discovered thiamine, also known as vitamin B_1. Beriberi became widespread in the southern United States after the adoption of "polished" rice, which was milled and stripped of the rice bran and germ and, consequently, vitamin B_1.

Over the next few years, the vitamins A, C, D, and E were discovered. As scientists learned more about these nutrients and their role in optimum health, the government encouraged Americans to eat more calories from a wide variety of foods. The US Department of Agriculture (USDA) evolved to serve two distinct roles: to promote farm products by getting Americans to eat more food, and to educate the citizenry about proper nutrition. These roles were complementary at a time when the majority of the citizenry needed to simply eat more to make up for widespread nutritional deficiencies. In 1917, the USDA released its first general recommendations for healthy eating, called "How to Select Foods." Food was divided into five groups: milk and meat, cereals, vegetables and fruits, fats and fatty foods, and sugars and sugary food. This marked the beginning of a steady stream of nutritional advice by the USDA, advice that has changed constantly as science has made new discoveries.

TOP 100 REASONS TO AVOID PROCESSED FOODS

The ingredient list for Strawberry Fruit Roll-Ups doesn't include . . . strawberries.

With the benefit of hindsight, we can see that many of the government's dietary recommendations haven't worked. The more the message has changed (margarine or butter?), the more confusing the advice became. And for the average American it's getting more confusing each and every day.

We hope to clear up much of this confusion by reestablishing the wisdom of whole foods. So let's travel back to our number one Bad Mood Food.

Our Insatiable Appetite for Sugar

It might be surprising to hear, but sugar is a relatively new food in our diet. For the vast majority of human existence no one had access to this sweet substance. But over the course of the last 500 years we've slowly consumed more and more, until we now find it in nearly every processed food in the grocery store.

Sugar goes by dozens and dozens of different names. But the ancient inhabitants of Mesopotamia and China had no word for it. It was first discovered in sugarcane in the South Pacific, and its use slowly migrated to Asia and the Indian subcontinent. Sugar was so difficult to come by during the Middle Ages that the king of England, Henry III, once ordered three pounds of sugar with the caveat "If so much could be had at one time." Today the average American eats three pounds of sugar every week.

Much of the colonization of the Western Hemisphere surrounded the cultivation of sugar. Eventually European sea powers like Portugal and

TOP 100 REASONS TO AVOID PROCESSED FOODS

The ingredient list for low-fat Dannon Fruit on the Bottom strawberry yogurt does contain strawberries . . . followed by sugar, fructose syrup, fructose, and high fructose corn syrup.

Spain began to cultivate sugarcane off the African coast on islands like São Tomé and the Canary Islands. These were the first slave plantations— the model for what would turn the Lesser and Greater Antilles of the Caribbean Sea into the Sugar Islands.

Spain's plantations started on modern-day Cuba (sugarcane, of course, was introduced by Columbus). Over time, more than 7 million Africans, shackled in slave boats, made the journey across the Middle Passage to work the sugarcane fields of the Sugar Islands in order to feed the modern world's fledgling sweet tooth.

When Americans learn about slaves in school, we hear about those who tended to the cotton and tobacco fields of the South, but the nexus of the slave trade economy was sugar. The British, French, Spanish, Dutch, and Portuguese all had large populations of slaves producing sugar in the Caribbean. It was undoubtedly the most difficult and feared form of indentured work. Harvesting sugarcane meant stooping down and swinging a heavy machete at the base of a reed thousands of times a day in suffocating humidity and baking heat. Contemporary Americans worry about blood diamonds, but throughout the eighteenth and nineteenth centuries, we lamented about "blood sugar," when a pound of sugar was said to cost two pounds of African flesh.

After losing significant sugarcane holdings in the West Indies, the French emperor Napoleon Bonaparte turned with fervor to the sugar beet. He understood that if Parisians were deprived of their new favorite source of calories, he'd likely face an uprising. Sugar had been extracted from beets before but never as a reliable source of sugar for large popula-

13

TOP 100 REASONS TO AVOID PROCESSED FOODS

The vegetable oils found in many processed foods are high in inflammatory omega-6 fatty acids that are linked to depression, heart disease, and diabetes.

TOP 100 REASONS TO AVOID PROCESSED FOODS

Tropicana Peach Orchard Punch is only 5 percent juice and has more high fructose corn syrup than soda.

14

tions. Napoleon established six laboratories and devoted 80,000 acres to the task. Soon France was producing enough sugar domestically that the emperor blocked all cane sugar imports. Once Europe gained sugar independence, the movement to abolish slavery gained serious momentum.

By 1910, about 800,000 acres of beets were grown in California, Colorado, and Nebraska. Beet sugar and cane sugar share about equal parts of the American sugar supply. Labor costs to process beet sugar are much lower than those to produce cane sugar, but sugarcane owners have a lot of political pull that protects their industry. Both industries will no doubt coexist for years to come, but the biggest threat to their long-term market share is plentiful, cheap sweeteners made from corn—cornstarch, glucose, maltodextrin, dextrose, crystalline fructose, sorbitol, mannitol, corn syrup solids, and high fructose corn syrup (HCFS). Recently, the Corn Refiners Association asked the FDA to change the name of high fructose corn syrup to corn sugar.

AMERICAN SUGAR CONSUMPTION PER YEAR

1700—5 pounds per person

1800—23 pounds per person

1900—70 pounds per person

2000—152 pounds per person (52 teaspoons per day)

When you see those numbers, you wonder how such an increase took place. But the case of a southern doctor named John Pemberton is illustrative of how this happened. We'd argue he's likely responsible for more sugar calories being consumed in America than any other human being.

TOP 100 REASONS TO AVOID PROCESSED FOODS

A nine-ounce container of Wise Nacho Cheese Dip contains twelve grams of trans fats.

Pemberton got his medical degree at the Southern Botanico Medical College in Georgia in 1850. He received additional training as a pharmacist and settled in Columbus, Georgia, where he worked as a druggist. During the Civil War he joined the Confederate Army and was shot at the Battle of Columbus. Like many wounded soldiers of the day, the pharmacist became addicted to the painkiller morphine. He settled in Atlanta at the conclusion of hostilities and developed an elixir to cure his addiction, calling it Pemberton's French Wine of Coca, a mixture of French Bordeaux with extracts of the coca leaf and kola nut. When Atlanta outlawed the sale of alcohol, Pemberton had to reformulate, swapping sugar water for wine and calling his new medicinal brew Coca-Cola.

In 1915 the iconic contoured glass bottle held 6.5 ounces. After World War II it increased to 10 ounces, and a 26-ounce "family-size" container was introduced as well. By 1960 the aluminum can was introduced and ounces-per-serving increased to 12—that's about 10 teaspoons worth of sugar. Then came the 1970s and the 2-liter plastic bottles, upping the "family size." In the '80s self-service fountain drinks were introduced and convenience stores across the country began selling 32- and 44-ounce individual servings branded as "Thirstbuster" and "Big Gulp." A few years later the 20-ounce plastic bottle had all but replaced the Coke can, and in 2009 Coca-Cola launched its advertising campaign "Open Happiness," which is ironic considering how much havoc this beverage can wreak on your mental health if it's abused, which is happening on a massive scale. Today it's estimated that the average American drinks more than 600 twelve-ounce sodas a year!

Why Everyone Got So Confused about Fat

The next biggest change to our diet is the inclusion of processed vegetable oils. Prior to the industrial revolution humans didn't have a way to process large amounts of oil from things like cottonseed and safflower. You might be surprised to learn what our staple dietary fats were before these cheap, factory-made oils entered our food supply.

Before highways and before railroads, America conducted her commerce via steamship over water through a system of rivers, canals, and lakes. In the 1800s, Cincinnati was the heart of the developed United States. At the time it was known to the world as Porkopolis. That's because not so long ago, the most widely consumed meat in this nation was swine.

This was before refrigeration. The biggest enemy of nineteenth-century butchers was spoilage. Eating cows didn't make a whole lot of sense: Distributing the meat of a freshly killed 1,500-pound animal before it went bad was difficult without roads and temperature-controlled trains. But pigs are fatty, which makes them excellent for salt curing because they don't lose flavor.

Cincinnati is on the Ohio River, which flows to the Mississippi River, which leads to the ever-important port of New Orleans. From the mouth of the mighty Mississippi, Porkopolis distributed meat throughout the coastal southern United States. The by-products of pork production meant that the burgeoning metropolis was also home to many tanneries, boot

TOP 100 REASONS TO AVOID PROCESSED FOODS

16

Every time you buy a processed food like soy milk or a Wendy's hamburger, you support Monsanto, the infamous multinational corporation that created Agent Orange (and nearly caused the extinction of the bald eagle with the production of the pesticide DDT). That's because Monsanto now controls more than 90 percent of the soybean market.

TOP 100 REASONS TO AVOID PROCESSED FOODS

Animal feed given to factory-farmed cows contains rendered roadkill, euthanized cats and dogs, and plastic pellets as a cheap form of "roughage."

makers, and upholsters. Animal fats were hot commodities, as they were rendered and molded into soap and candles. Breaking down pigs was a highly efficient process and known as the disassembly line—an idea that would later be reverse-engineered by Henry Ford to produce automobiles.

A major economic depression in the 1870s caused two important citizens of Porkopolis to join forces in order to cut costs and survive the bear market. They formed a company that would eventually be responsible for the greatest dietary shift in our country's history. William Procter brought his candle-making business to the states after a fire destroyed his business in England. James Gamble fled Ireland during the Great Potato Famine and became a soap manufacturer. In a twist of fate, the two men happened to marry sisters in Cincinnati. Together, the brothers-in-law formed Procter & Gamble, a soap- and candle-manufacturing operation.

At the time, soap was sold in huge wheels that were sliced into custom-sized portions at general stores. Procter and Gamble decided to take a chance by mass-producing individually wrapped bars of soap. To pull this off, the brother-in-laws needed to drastically reduce the price of their raw ingredients, which meant finding a replacement for expensive animal fats. They settled on a mix of palm and coconut oils and created the first soap that floated in water—a handy invention when clothes and dishes alike were washed in a sudsy basin. Hard pressed to come up with a name for this new product, Procter looked to the bible for inspiration and found it in Psalm 45:8: "All thy garments smell of myrrh, and aloes, and cassia, out of the ivory palaces, whereby they have made thee glad." The word *Ivory* was trademarked, and in short order Americans all over the country would know the purity of this soap.

Oddly enough, the company to thank for the fact that America now eats so much vegetable oil has never produced much in the way of food. Thanks to Procter & Gamble the United States boosted the production of a waste product of cotton farming, cottonseed oil. To ensure a steady, cheap supply for soap production the company formed a subsidiary in 1902 called Buckeye Cotton Oil Co. Before processing, cottonseed oil is cloudy red and bitter to the taste because of a natural phytochemical called gossypol (it's used today in China as male birth control) and is toxic to most animals, causing dangerous spikes in the body's potassium levels, organ damage, and paralysis.

An issue of *Popular Science* from the era sums up the evolution of cottonseed nicely: "What was garbage in 1860 was fertilizer in 1870, cattle feed in 1880, and table food and many things else in 1890." But it entered our food supply slowly. It wasn't until a new food-processing invention of hydrogenation that cottonseed oil found its way into the kitchens of America's restaurants and homes.

Edwin Kayser, a German chemist, wrote to Procter & Gamble on October 18, 1907, about a new chemical process that could create a solid fat from a liquid. The company's researchers had been interested in producing a solid form of cottonseed oil for years, and Kayser described his new process as "of the greatest possible importance to soap manufacturers." The company purchased US rights to the patents and created a lab on the Procter & Gamble campus, known as Ivorydale, to experiment with the new technology. Soon the company's scientists produced a new creamy, pearly white substance out of cottonseed oil. It looked a lot like the most popular cooking fat of the day: lard. Before long, Procter & Gamble sold this new substance (known today as hydrogenated

---

TOP 100 REASONS TO AVOID PROCESSED FOODS　　18

Nature's Path Organic Crunchy Vanilla Sunrise gluten-free cereal is sweetened with organic evaporated cane juice and organic inulin— fancy ways to say sugar.

vegetable oil) to home cooks as a replacement for animal fats.

Procter & Gamble filed a patent application for the new creation in 1910, describing it as "a food product consisting of a vegetable oil, preferably cottonseed oil, partially hydrogenated, and hardened to a homogeneous white or yellowish semi-solid closely resembling lard. The special object of the invention is to provide a new food product for a shortening in cooking." They came up with the name "Crisco"—which they thought conjured up crispness, freshness, and cleanliness.

Convincing homemakers to swap butter and lard for a new fat created in a factory would be quite a task, so the new form of food needed a new marketing strategy. Never before had Procter & Gamble—or any company for that matter—put so much marketing support or advertising dollars behind a product. They hired the J. Walter Thompson Agency, America's first full-service advertising agency staffed by real artists and professional writers. Samples of Crisco were mailed to grocers, restaurants, nutritionists, and home economists. Eight alternative marketing strategies were tested in different cities and their impacts calculated and compared. Doughnuts were fried in Crisco and handed out in the streets. Women who purchased the new industrial fat got a free cookbook of Crisco recipes. It opened with the line, "The culinary world is revising its entire cookbook on account of the advent of Crisco, a new and altogether different cooking fat." Recipes for asparagus soup, baked salmon with Colbert sauce, stuffed beets, curried cauliflower, and tomato sandwiches all called for three to four tablespoons of Crisco.

Health claims on food packaging were then unregulated, and the copywriters claimed that cottonseed oil was healthier than animal fats for digestion. Advertisements in the *Ladies' Home Journal* encouraged homemakers

TOP 100 REASONS TO AVOID PROCESSED FOODS

Lay's Light and Pringles Light potato chips contain olestra, a fat substitute that leaches fat-soluble nutrients like vitamin D from the body and causes diarrhea, bloating, and "anal leakage."

to try the new fat and "realize why its discovery will affect every family in America." The unprecedented product rollout resulted in the sales of 2.6 million pounds of Crisco in 1912 and 60 million pounds just four years later. This new food bolstered the bottom line of a company whose other products were Ivory Soap, Lenox Soap, White Naphtha Laundry Soap, and Star Soap. It also helped usher in the age of margarine as well as low-fat foods.

Procter & Gamble's claims about Crisco touching the lives of every American proved eerily prescient. The substance (like many of its imitators) was 50 percent trans fat, and it wasn't until the 1990s that its health risks were understood. It is estimated that for every 2 percent increase in consumption of trans fat (still found in many processed and fast foods) the risk of heart disease increases by 23 percent. As you'll learn throughout this book, and as surprising as it might be to hear, the fact that animal fats pose this same risk is not supported by science.

The Facts on Cholesterol

It's important to note that the mid-twentieth century was a time when many of our problems were solved by silver-bullet solutions. The atom bomb ended the war. Polio was cured with a vaccine. And by this time it was clear that a lot of upper-class men were dying from a new form of heart disease. Soon the hunt was on for a cure, and with all good intentions we became a nation obsessed with dietary cholesterol and fat.

"Fatal coronary event" became an official diagnosis recognized by the *International Classification of Diseases* manual in 1948, and that same year

Congress established the National Heart Institute to study the phenomenon that Florida's Senator Claude Pepper claimed was "far more dangerous than Hitler." The majority of men afflicted with this new disease had plaques in their arteries made of cholesterol, calcium, and inflammatory cells called macrophages, and when these deposits became inflamed and broke off, they sometimes blocked coronary arteries and caused a heart attack.

A physiologist named Ancel Keys established the Laboratory of Physiological Hygiene at the University of Minnesota, where he performed many of the world's first diet studies. He also started the first study of cardiac disease that followed research subjects' diet and lifestyle into the future. Like other doctors of the day, Keys was intrigued by this new disease that mainly affected rich white men. He enlisted 281 businessmen from Minneapolis, making sure to include Governor Edward Thye and coach Bernie Bierman of the five-time national champion University of Minnesota football team. Every year, the men arrived at Keys's lab underneath the football stadium for a full physical exam. A blood sample was taken to measure total cholesterol, along with a urine sample, an EKG, a chest X-ray, and measures of body fat and blood pressure. Keys was eager to prove a relatively new theory that dietary fat caused heart disease by raising blood cholesterol.

Keys turned his attention to a large-scale epidemiological study of heart disease in Finland and Japan. He compared the diet of the Finns, who had one of the highest rates of heart disease in the world, with that of the Japanese, who had one of the lowest incidences of heart disease. Finns were known for eating a high-fat diet that famously included spreading butter over cheese, while the Japanese were known for eating

TOP 100 REASONS TO AVOID PROCESSED FOODS

Old El Paso Taco Dinner kits contain ethoxyquin, a chemical invented by Monsanto in the 1950s and originally registered as a pesticide. There is very limited human safety data, but in a test tube it damages the DNA of human immune cells.

prodigious amounts of fresh seafood. This work eventually led to a now extremely controversial paper called the Six Countries Study that looked at the correlation between total average fat intake and death from heart disease in Australia, Canada, England, Italy, Japan, and the United States. Keys's findings were unmistakable and showed a perfect correlation between dietary fat in populations and deaths from heart disease.

Today we know that Keys's data were seriously flawed. If it had been accurately named, the study would have been known as the Twenty-Two Countries Study—Keys analyzed the data from that many nations and then chose the six countries he needed to prove his theory.

If Keys had included all twenty-two countries in his study, the correlation between dietary fat and heart disease would have disappeared. If he had used six different populations—such as the Masai in Kenya, who mainly drink milk and cow's blood, and the Inuit, who subsist almost solely on fatty arctic sea life—the conclusion would have reversed itself and the graph would have shown that the more fat populations eat, the less heart disease they suffer.

Nevertheless, Keys's paper was immensely compelling. He would go on to appear on the cover of *Time* magazine as "Mr. Cholesterol." And then, on September 23, 1955, something happened that cemented Keys's theories in the American mind for several generations to come.

The Heart Attack Heard 'round America

The summer of 1955 had been stressful for President Dwight Eisenhower. His approval rating was 79 percent, but behind the scenes, the president was worrying his personal physician, Major General Howard Snyder.

Although Eisenhower had quit his four-pack-a-day smoking habit a few years before, he'd recently been exploding in fits of red-faced, vein-bulging rage at his longtime secretary for minor mishaps. A vacation was overdue, and the president and his wife, Mamie, flew to Denver, where they'd been married three decades earlier.

Eisenhower started the morning of September 23 by writing to Lyndon Johnson, the Senate majority leader, chiding him to refrain from "living life to the hilt" too soon after Johnson's July heart attack. The president then hit a round of golf at the Cherry Hills Country Club. After eating a burger loaded with Bermuda onions for lunch, the president stopped golfing due to indigestion. He returned to the house and worked on a painting, then took a light dinner with friends and family and retired to bed early. Around one in the morning, the president awoke with what he thought was severe heartburn. Mamie called the doctor, and when he arrived Ike was pale and sweaty. The doctor dosed him with morphine. An electrocardiographic examination confirmed the doctor's fears: The president had survived a massive heart attack. The medical team in Denver summoned the country's leading cardiologist at the time, Paul White, who had already treated some of the wealthiest heart disease patients of the era: Andrew Carnegie, William Randolph Hearst, and Cornelius Vanderbilt.

Within the next year, the American Heart Association embraced the idea that excess fat and cholesterol in the diet—Ike's burger—was causing the epidemic of heart disease. The association launched the Prudent Diet, which recommended swapping butter, meat, and dairy for vegetables and vegetable oils. Forty years after the invention of Crisco, a major medical organization had endorsed it for the first time as a preventative for heart disease. It would be nearly half a century before the AHA reversed course

TOP 100 REASONS TO AVOID PROCESSED FOODS

There are more than eighty ingredients in one Oscar Mayer Lunchables Breaded Chicken and Mozzarella sandwich.

and advised against eating vegetable oils that were hydrogenated because they actually cause heart disease rather than prevent it.

The president's cardiologist helped Ancel Keys get funding for a follow-up to the Six Countries Study, which would be become the Seven Countries Study. At the time, Keys's follow-up was the biggest epidemiological study ever conducted, following more than 12,000 men between the ages of 40 and 49. This study had the same fundamental problem as the one that preceded it: Keys selected countries that would support his hypothesis. And thus we got stuck with the false message that fat was bad.

What Does It All Mean?

It seems like it's all so simple, right? We're eating too much sugar and vegetable fats—a diet that's predisposing us to not only obesity and diabetes but all kinds of mental disorders. We should just make a switch and we'll be all good, right? That's not how the food industry works. Instead, they want to forever solve our problems with more technology rather than by returning to traditional ways of eating that previously prevented all the epidemic diseases our country now faces.

Animal fat—the kind that doesn't come from factory-farm animals eating unnatural diets—is anything but unhealthy for the human body. It's what we've been subsisting on for tens of thousands of years. It's what your body was designed to eat. But public awareness of this simple fact remains obscured by the MAD system of food production.

By 2006, a clear link was established between heart disease and the type of trans fats found in Crisco, margarine, and much processed food and fast food. And in 2011, a study showed that consuming trans fats greatly increases the risk of clinical depression. The National Academy of Sciences states that no level of trans fats in food is safe. The FDA requires the amount of this deadly substance to be listed on food labels, but, unfortunately, it allows food manufacturers to claim "zero trans fats" if a product contains less than half a gram per serving. So if you happen to eat an entire bag of potato chips (or any combination of everyday American snack foods), you can easily enter the unsafe range of consumption of trans fat, even though all the packages claim "zero" levels of the substance.

Aside from the fact that these fats increase the risk of heart disease, new science shows that they also cross the placenta and may compromise brain development in the fetus. Studies show that the more trans fats a pregnant woman eats, the lower her baby's birth weight. And the more trans fats in a woman's blood, the greater her risk of breast cancer.

After the alarm sounded on trans fats, food processors raced to find a safe alternative. But rather than return to traditional fats that humans have been eating for thousands of years, the food industry turned to a MAD solution: fatty acid randomization. This process turns fully hydrogenated vegetable fats into saturated fats. Technically, it's known as interesterification, and that's the term you'll see on food labels.

Food processors are now able to take partially hydrogenated vegetable oils (like margarine and Crisco) and fully hydrogenate them to get rid of trans fats, producing yet another new fat never before consumed by humans. Just as there were no health studies on trans fats prior to their domination of the food supply starting in 1912, no studies of long-term effects of interesterified fats have been conducted, either.

Early research, however, offers serious causes for concern. Interestified fats raise blood sugar by 20 percent and also increase blood insulin (telling your body to store fat). They appear to shift cholesterol levels to unhealthy ratios of "good" HDL and "bad" LDL cholesterol. While it will be decades before the full health effects of these fats are known, one thing is for certain: When you partake of the Modern American Diet, you are always an unwilling and unknowing test subject for manufactured food products that have unknown and unstudied effects on the human body.

Does that sound like the road to happiness?

Now that we know how unnatural the foods are that make up the MAD diet, it's time to take a look at how we can reverse course.

3

Bad Food, Bad Mood

At first, maybe you have trouble staying focused. Or perhaps you don't have as much energy as you used to. It could be that you're more thirsty than usual. Then again, maybe you are experiencing a persistent low mood. Strong fluctuations in appetite are another symptom, as are frequent trips to the bathroom. You're easily irritated lately.

These symptoms might feel like the normal ups and downs of your body, or perhaps indicators of advancing age. But the reality is that you're experiencing the first signs of an illness that is striking America in epidemic proportions. It's an illness that leads directly to the most common causes of premature death and that at first was known only as syndrome X. If syndrome X proceeds, it will lead to weight gain, diabetes, heart disease, stroke, cancer, and a host of mental problems, including depression and Alzheimer's disease. Today, syndrome X is better known as metabolic syndrome, and it's caused by the food we're eating: the Modern American Diet (MAD).

We can point fingers—large, faceless, multinational corporations; government subsidies; and a populace that's ever more removed from food production each day. But the fact is that our food supply has changed more in the past 100 years than it had in the previous 100,000. It's clear to many that our diet makes us fat and predisposed to suffer from the most common causes of death. What is often overlooked is how our food choices impact brain function. The MAD choices we make promote low moods, reduce our ability to focus, and increase our risk of the most common mental illnesses.

We'll look through these changes individually in this chapter and highlight the worst practices, the common culprits, that are collectively tanking our mood.

The first and most important dietary change is the amount of sugar we're eating, as well as other foods that our body immediately turns into simple sugars. The other massive change is that we've switched from animal fats to eating industrial fats produced from corn and soy. In the last one hundred years, we've swapped small family farms for a factory-farm model of agriculture. This means both less diversity in the nutrients that we eat as well as a system of farming that relies on pesticides, hormones, and antibiotics.

But those aren't the only toxins in our MAD food supply, as you'll soon see.

Mood Buster #1: Sugar and Refined Carbs

Over the course of the past two hundred years, we've increased our sugar intake by 3,000 percent. This is the biggest single change to the human diet since the invention of fire. In the year 1800, Americans ate about five pounds of sugar per person a year. One hundred years later, our sugar consumption was at seventy pounds per year. Today, the average American consumes around 150 pounds of sugar and sweeteners per year, according to the USDA—we're eating as much sugar *every week* as we used to eat annually.

Sugar is today understood to be the primary driving force for the obesity

TOP 100 REASONS TO AVOID PROCESSED FOODS

The hidden costs of the dollar menu at fast-food chains are steep. The annual expense of medical care and missed work add up to $83 billion for depression, $183 billion for Alzheimer's disease, $270 billion for obesity, and $174 billion for diabetes.

TOP 100 REASONS TO AVOID PROCESSED FOODS

While the cause of migraine headaches is still largely unknown, many migraine patients report fewer headaches after the removal of monosodium glutamate (MSG) from their diet.

epidemic. When journalist Gary Taubes pulled together thousands of research articles for his book *Why We Get Fat*, the answer was strikingly clear—sugar and refined carbohydrates. And even if you manage to stay skinny on the MAD, science increasingly suggests you will suffer from sugar's ill effects.

Studies show that countries with the highest per capita intake of sugar are the countries with the highest rates of depression. Eating MAD amounts of sugar also increases the risk of dementia. Experts now even propose calling some types of Alzheimer's disease "diabetes type 3." Others wonder if some forms of clinical depression should be considered "metabolic syndrome type 2." This means that the foods that are responsible for heart disease, cancer, and diabetes are also responsible for something else: our most common brain disorders.

Eating so much sugar actually shrinks your brain. Diets high in sugar (or refined carbohydrates) decrease brain-derived neurotrophic factor, also known as BDNF, a chemical we discussed in Chapter 1, that helps your brain to grow and produce new brain cells.

Studies show that high blood sugar, the frequent consequence of a sugary diet, leads to a smaller hippocampus and amygdala. These are the regions of your brain that help regulate mood, memory, anxiety, and cognition. Part of the reason we enjoy sugar so much is because its presence signals to our brains that we're eating a safe form of energy. Your tastebuds have only one receptor for sweetness but two dozen for bitterness. Plants protect themselves from predators by developing an arsenal of chemical weapons. Bitter compounds are what the natural world uses to warn us of poison—a plant's defense from being eaten. Our ability to taste these bitter compounds is ten thousand times greater than our ability to taste sweetness.

Carbage In, Nutrients Out

The word *sugar* is synonymous with carbohydrate. All plants are constructed of sugars, and popularly we know these as complex carbohydrates. So whether we're talking about romaine lettuce or oats or asparagus, these are all complex carbohydrates. The opposite, of course, are known as simple carbohydrates or simple sugars. These are plants that have been refined and processed to create things like pasta, bread, pizza dough, and fruit juice. Collectively, we refer to these foods as "carbage,"* or carbohydrate garbage. They make up the majority of calories in the MAD lifestyle. Whether it comes in the form of soda or pasta, carbage is one of the main dietary culprits behind America's uptick in weight and downtick in happiness. Your body knows when you've eaten your fill of whole foods. Carbage is so new to our diet that our bodies don't have off switches to tell our brains when we've eaten enough of these simple sugars—but protein, fat, and complex carbohydrates have these "switches." When we eat meats, dairy, and whole vegetables, they tell our digestive and nervous systems that we've had enough and should stop eating.

We've all heard with an almost religious fervor about how bad fats are, but we're not told that when we eat fat, our gallbladder releases the hormone cholecystokinin that instructs our brain to stop eating when we're full. This simple fact explains why people are able to eat a pile of pancakes but couldn't do the same with bacon. Proteins in food cause our stomach to release the hormone called peptide YY that tells our body we're satiated so that it doesn't become overwhelmed by too much of this macronutrient. Complex carbohydrates are tough to break down, and they expand our stomach proportionally, alerting the brain via the vagus nerve that we literally can't eat anymore.

One of the most fundamental problems in the MAD is that carbage is absorbed in the first two feet of our intestines, before our brains can recog-

---

* We'd like to thank both Nina Planck and Jimmy Moore (he lost 180 pounds!) for bringing this very apt term to our attention.

TOP 100 REASONS TO AVOID PROCESSED FOODS

Researchers found that kids who eat a junk-food diet are most likely to have behavioral problems at age 7.

nize how much we've eaten. So we continue eating calories, which get stored as fat. That's because high blood sugar puts our body in fat-storing mode.

The fact that we have no problem—and even enjoy—overeating refined carbohydrates is why we're lured into convenience stores with advertisements of free soda refills and into restaurants with all-you-can-eat pasta buffets. The fact that fat and protein are filling is why steak restaurants challenge customers to eat supersize cuts of meat—like a seventy-six-ounce rib eye in under an hour—and offer free meals if customers do so. (If they don't, of course, they pay in full.) Vegan restaurants would have just as much success if they challenged customers to eat seventy-six ounces of asparagus. Either task is nearly impossible.

Need a Fix?

While many of us have trouble resisting a platter of cookies or a bowl of chips, it's unlikely that you know anyone who regularly goes on broccoli benders. Not surprisingly, it's becoming clear to scientists that simple sugars are addictive. Eating sweet things causes the same changes in the area of our brains that regulates pleasure and reward (the nucleus accumbens) that lights up with the use of cocaine and heroin.

In studies at Princeton University's Neuroscience Institute, Bart Hoebel, PhD, has found that rats taken off high-sugar diets experience the hallmark symptoms of drug withdrawal: chattering teeth, severe anxiety, and an unwillingness to explore new surroundings. Moreover, when these animals are reintroduced to sugar, neurotransmitters like dopamine increase, just as they do in the brains of drug addicts who are reintroduced to heroin. Hoebel's research has also shown that rodent brains actually prefer sugar over cocaine. To translate these findings to humans, researchers used functional magnetic resonance imaging to scan the brains of subjects shown images of sugary foods. They found that the pictures activate those same areas that fired in the brains of rats eating the sugary foods. And speaking of addictive substances, you might be surprised to know that the number-one additive in cigarettes is . . . sugar. Researchers speculate that the sugars in alcohol (metabolized by the body much like carbage) is part of what makes it addictive.

Why Sugar Makes You Sick, Fat, and Unhappy

The scientific name for table sugar is *sucrose*. It's actually made up of two individual sugars—glucose and fructose—in a 50/50 ratio. Let's talk about the first one: glucose.

Every cell in your body can absorb glucose and use it as fuel. When people refer to "blood sugar," they're talking about glucose. It dissolves in your blood and transports energy throughout your body. Your body regulates the amount of glucose in your blood with the two hormones insulin and glucagon. The pancreas releases both. Normally, your body maintains blood sugar in a narrow range to avoid hypoglycemia (low blood sugar) and hyperglycemia (high blood sugar), both of which can cause serious health problems.

When your blood sugar is low, you get agitated and irritable—something you likely experienced the last time you went too long without eating. You can also experience the effects of low blood sugar after eating a meal high in refined carbohydrates. These foods spike your blood sugar level for a while. As your body reacts, it then crashes down—especially for individuals with a condition called reactive hypoglycemia. As a result, you might have trouble concentrating, feel lethargic, or sink into a bad mood.

The opposite of low blood sugar is hyperglycemia. This means there is too much sugar in your blood, and it's a condition that damages arteries and helps promote development of arterial plaques (which can rupture, triggering a heart attack or stroke). High blood sugar ages our blood vessels and over time shrinks our brains, damages our vision and nerves, and is associated with an increased risk of developing depression and Alzheimer's disease.

When sugar enters your bloodstream, the pancreas releases the hormone insulin, which signals your cells to absorb sugar, which then fuels activities like reading the words on this page. Glucose is also used to build muscle, remove toxins, and repair DNA. Once your immediate energy needs are met, insulin tells your body to store excess glucose as glycogen in your liver and muscles. Once these stores are filled, insulin directs your body to store any excess sugar as fat. These fat molecules are called triglycerides, and they accumulate around the belly in men and around the hips and buttocks in women.

As we eat more sugar, we release more insulin. But over time, the accumulation of fat changes hormonal signaling and the body begins to ignore insulin. This condition is called insulin resistance. When the body stops recognizing this hormone, more sugar accumulates in the blood; in response, the pancreas releases even more insulin. Soon the body is swimming in too much sugar and too much insulin. This is what is known as diabetes, and it speeds the aging of the brain. More on that soon.

The second sugar, fructose, is found in small amounts in ripe fruit. But the majority of fructose in our diet does not come from fruit but from refined sugar and high fructose corn syrup, or HFCS. Because we eat too much of these added sugars in our MADness, we're consequently eating too much fructose.

Our liver converts fructose into triglycerides that, when we eat this

---

TOP 100 REASONS TO AVOID PROCESSED FOODS

Excess antibiotics use by factory farms is largely to blame for the development of superbugs like MRSA, a flesh-eating bacteria that kills eighteen thousand Americans a year.

sugar in excess, accumulate around our internal organs. The resultant layer of fat—called visceral fat—increases our risk of developing heart disease and many types of cancer. Visceral fat appears to produce inflammation associated with insulin resistance. Another by-product of turning fructose into fat is uric acid, which constricts the blood vessels in your arteries and causes high blood pressure.

Fructose boosts production of a recently recognized type of LDL cholesterol called "small dense LDL cholesterol" (sdLDL) that elevates the risk of heart disease. SdLDL is the same type of cholesterol that's produced when you eat trans fats found in processed foods. It gets worse. Fructose shuts down your satiety hormone, leptin, and turns on your hunger hormone, ghrelin. It's a little trick that plants invented to get us to eat more fruit and spread more of their seeds. That's why it's so easy to drink soda without getting full.

We're all told as children to not eat too many sweets because they'll rot our teeth, but no one takes the time to explain why this is so. Two types of bacteria in our mouths, mutans streptococci and lactobacilli, thrive off sugar. The waste product of their sugar consumption—literally their excrement—is an acidic solution that destroys the enamel of our teeth. Cavities were extremely rare among primitive cultures like the African Bantu and the Yup'ik Eskimos of Kipnuk, Alaska, but that changed as soon as carbage became part of their diet.

Traditional societies also don't typically have acne, a skin problem that affects 95 percent of teenagers in the Western world. Both the Kitavans of Papua New Guinea and Ache hunter-gatherers of Paraguay, for example, don't eat any sugar or refined carbohydrates and are blemish free. Too much sugar triggers the production of androgens, male hormones that promote the excretion of a greasy substance called sebum that clogs pores. In addition, sugar helps promote cyst formation inside women's ovaries, a disease known as polycystic ovary disease. It's one of the leading causes of infertility and affects more than 10 percent of American women.

Why French Fries Cause Wrinkles and Shrink Your Brain

Eating MAD amounts of sugar and refined carbohydrates speeds up the aging of the human body. When our blood becomes too high in glucose, sugar begins to randomly attach to the proteins in our tissues through a process known as glycation. This is the same process that browns foods, such as bread crust. The more carbage we eat, the more glycation occurs. The most visible signs of glycation are deep wrinkles. Sugar attaches to collagen and cross-links the tissue, decreasing flexibility. As the skin hardens, it loses elasticity and wrinkles form. Doctors have compared the process of glycation to tanning leather. Glycation promotes the formation of sugar-coated proteins called advanced glycation end products (AGEs); these AGEs promote inflammation and further advance aging by releasing free radicals that destroy our cells and DNA. Some plaques that form in the brains of Alzheimer's patients are made of AGEs. These molecules inflame and shrink the hippocampus, the part of our brain that forms memories. Thanks to brain-imaging studies, we now know that people with chronic high blood sugar have shrunken hippocampuses.

Inflammation is a popular word today in medicine. This process is now linked to brain disorders like depression and dementia, as well as heart disease, cancer, and diabetes. As we eat more and more sugar, one root of this inflammation seems apparent. Cancer cells thrive on sugar, and that's why it's no surprise that high blood sugar is linked to the formation of at least twenty-four different kinds of cancer, such as that of the pancreas, breast, liver, uterus, rectum, bladder, and colon. In addition to insulin, dietary sugar causes an increased production of insulin-like growth factors (IGFs), which is strongly correlated with the ability of cancers to spread. Women with high levels of IGFs are 50 percent more likely to develop breast cancer, and men with high levels are 65 percent more likely to develop prostate cancer.

The Centers for Disease Control and Prevention (CDC) estimates that seventy-nine million American adults are prediabetic. As patients with diabetes age, the long-term effects of unregulated high blood sugar become apparent. The lens of the eye becomes cloudy due the accumulation of AGEs, and vision is further impaired by damage to the optic nerve that runs from the eyeball to the brain. Half of men with diabetes can't get erections due to the damage of the small blood vessels of the penis. Kidneys get clogged with AGEs and stop working. Nerve damage also causes diabetics' feet and hands to go numb. The small arteries that deliver blood to the feet and toes slowly deteriorate from high blood sugar, and this poor circulation compromises the delivery of nutrients, antibiotics, and immune cells needed for wound healing. Eventually, the hands and feet rot. As the blood supply is compromised, doctors are left with few choices. Amputations start at the toes and work their way up the leg over the years. Blind, numb, impotent, depressed, memory impaired, dialysis dependent, wrinkled, and prematurely aged—the course of untreated diabetes makes it clear that sugar rots more than your teeth.

Mood Buster #2: Industrial Fats

We know that last section on sugar was tough, but we needed to show you the stark truth behind its consumption so as to help break its stranglehold on your health and mental well-being. Now, before we get to the good mood foods, we have to tell you about a few more important shifts in the American diet.

You've likely heard of omega-3s. They're constantly making the news for their ability to improve mood and protect against heart disease. But you might not know about a second set of fatty acids that are just as important as the omega-3s. They're called omega-6s and, like sugar, they represent much too large a portion of our MAD lifestyles.

Common sources of omega-6s include most of the vegetable oils found in convenience foods that come from corn, cottonseed, safflower, sunflower, and soy. These are what food processors use to make many foods that until very recently didn't even exist.

One industrial product made from these vegetable oils is margarine. The containers carry claims that they're heart healthy, but there's barely anything recognizable as food on their ingredient lists. Most varieties are made from a blend of new vegetable oils like soybean oil and canola oil and additives like soy lecithin, gelatin, and mono- and diglycerides (emulsifiers often derived from soy).

In fact, throughout the past one hundred years, for many Americans margarine was the top source of trans fat, a man-made substance created in vegetable oil processing that is now known to greatly increase your risk of depression and heart disease. New to our bodies, these fats have a different shape than natural fats; once incorporated into our cells, they essentially act like sand in our biochemical gears, promoting heart disease, diabetes, obesity, infertility, and Alzheimer's disease.

Both omega-3s and omega-6s are essential to our diet, and without them we'd die. Think about these two as the yin and yang of fats. Omega-6s are used to make signals that promote inflammation, while omega-3s give rise to signals that cool inflammation. They actually compete with each other for space in our cell membranes, like siblings sharing a bedroom. And they compete for the same regulatory enzymes, which means that increasing your omega-3 intake will be most effective if you also decrease the omega-6s in your diet.

Achieve a proper balance of these fats in the diet and you have a sharp, quick-thinking, mood-regulated brain. You'll have thin, silky blood that prevents inflammation and protects against brain disorders and heart disease. A diet too high in omega-6s—the MAD one—promotes blood more prone to clot and more likely to inflame the brain and cardiovascular system.

Nowhere is this imbalance more tilted toward omega-6s than in Israel, and it's responsible for what's known as the "Israeli paradox." Kosher laws forbid the consumption of cow flesh and milk products like butter at the same meal, and as the production of more soy and corn oil has spiked, practicing Jews have increasingly relied on vegetable oils to stay kosher in the modern world. And most likely thanks to omega-6s,

Israelis now have some of the lowest cholesterol levels of any Western country yet some of the highest rates of heart disease.

It's not just a matter of eating too many omega-6s oils in all our processed foods, we've also started feeding these foods to the animals we eat. Traditionally cows—and other ruminants such as sheep, goats, and bison—survived on a diet of grass. These animals salivate over a sun-drenched field of orchard grass, fescue, and red and white clover as a child does over different flavors of ice cream. Cows will pick an entire field clean of one grass (say, clover), and then start all over with their second favorite (say, millet). Not long ago, cows—much like fish today—and the products made from their milk (cheese, yogurt, butter) were quite good sources of omega-3s.

Today, most cows don't have access to grass and are fed a diet of soybeans and corn. Traditionally raised cattle fed an all-grass diet have a ratio of omega-6s to omega-3s that averages about 3 to 1. But the ratio of these fats in cattle fed soy and corn skews heavily in the direction of omega-6s: 20 to 1.

Chickens, too, used to live on the pasture, where they pecked away at grass and munched on grass-eating grubs. Their eggs contained abundant levels of these important fatty acids—how else do you power a young chick's brain? In fact, pastured-raised poultry produce eggs with a nearly perfect ratio of omega fats of 1 to 1. But sadly, today chickens, too, are fed a diet of corn and soy. Even farmed fish are now fed corn. One of the most MADly popular fish, tilapia, has an 11 to 1 ratio of omega-6s to omega-3s.

Mood Buster #3: How Our Meat Is "MADe"

Pork has been a staple of the human diet since Biblical times, and one reason is because pigs are incredibly efficient at recycling kitchen and garden scraps into usable protein. They also taste good.

To enhance the flavor of their meat, these animals were set out to pasture after the harvest to forge on things like acorns and peanuts. Often the meat was cured by hickory smoke and flavored with molasses and black pepper and aged for more than a year. (Southerners were notorious for eating bacon at every meal, like a condiment.) Before refrigeration, pigs were prized for their smaller size, making them easier to butcher and consume, and their fattier meat was perfect for salt curing (that's where the term "pork barrel" comes from—families used to survive on salted pork kept in a barrel during the winter).

These pasture-raised pigs were also a good source of vitamin D, a nutrient in which many Americans are now deficient. Not only that, but lard was the most popular cooking fat across the land—so those who ate it had a great source of vitamin D all winter long. (Steak was primarily eaten in places like New York City, where the cool climate prevented meat from spoiling quickly, and where there were large urban populations that could quickly devour a one-thousand-pound steer.)

Up until about a hundred years ago, Americans ate a wide variety of wild fowl, much in the same way we eat freely from the sea today. We ate roasted goose at Christmas, pies stuffed full of pigeon meat, roasted plover on toast, pheasant stew, and various birds that were eventually bred into what we now know as the modern, uniform, once-size-fits-all chicken. Not long ago, chicken was considered a luxury food. It was eaten mostly in the spring and summer when farmers culled their male birds (spring chickens). Hens were usually eaten in the winter and typically only after they'd passed their productive egg-laying years. As a result, their meat was tough, and so it was slow-cooked in soups or stews.

Change Isn't *Always* Good

Our livestock production has shifted from small farms and ranches into the hands of a small group of multinational corporations that control every step of meat production—as they say in the industry, from semen to cellophane. Large, vertically integrated companies control every step of food production from the breeding of cattle to the packing of hamburger meat.

The system has been described as an hourglass. At the top are a few million ranchers and cattle farmers. At the bottom are three hundred million consumers. At the bottleneck are a handful of corporations that make a profit off of every transaction. (Most Americans eat a ConAgra product every day, yet the majority of us have never heard of the company.) This system is built on efficiencies, and that means animals are produced in factories like any other commodity. Cheap factory meat is not nearly as healthy as the meat that comes from sustainably raised animals.

Animals forced to live such miserable lives have higher levels of stress hormones, which makes their meat tough and lowers concentrations of B-complex vitamins, zinc, copper, chromium, and vitamins A, E, and C. The stress of the modern slaughterhouse removes glycogen from muscles just before death, preventing the lactic acid buildup that makes for more tender meat. Meats without lactic acid buildup—factory-farmed meats— spoil more quickly and contain lower levels of antioxidants like glutathione, vitamin E, and superoxide dismutase and nutrients like potassium, zinc, iron, vitamin B_6, and linolenic acid—all things that are absolutely crucial for brain health, general well-being, and happiness.

Not long ago, the argument could be made that the fish counter was the last place in the grocery store where you could count on food being mostly wild-caught. That is no longer the case. Today many of our most popular fish, like salmon and tilapia, are farmed. Farmed fish contain a much lower concentration of omega-3s than do wild fish. Farmed fish are also higher in toxins like PCBs.

Cows are dosed with anabolic steroids so they can bulk up quickly for slaughter. Meat produced in this system is often laced with trace amounts of these drugs, and their long-term health effect on humans is unknown.

Pigs, too, are fed pharmaceuticals to speed growth, like the drug ractopamine, which makes pigs more aggressive and has been banned in at least 150 countries. If you're one of those people who think of Chinese products as inferior to American-made ones, you might be surprised to learn that China wouldn't import our pork for years because of speculation that ractopamine may cause heart problems and cancer in humans.

As with beef and pork, commoditizing chicken into a standard unit meant big changes in how the animals lived. Gone are the days of chickens running loose around the family farm eating a wide variety of nutrients in the form of bugs and grass. Their diet has been replaced by one of commodity grains, antibiotics, and growth promoters . . . and now those chemicals are being passed along to us, too.

Chicken get fed quite an interesting—and toxic—growth promoter: arsenic. It's believed that this poison prevents chickens from absorbing nutrients and that they overeat to make up for the deficiency. They reach market weight in forty days. This rate of growth is so unnatural that sometimes a bird's legs cannot support the weight of its girth and snap in half, at which point the birds are useless and are discarded. Like ractopamine, arsenic has been linked to heart disease and cancer (and is why, along with levels of chlorine, Russia wouldn't import US chicken for much of the last decade).

Through public service announcements, we've been warned about the dangers of not cooking meat thoroughly. This precaution is a direct result of the factory-farm system. The most notorious foodborne illness found at the meat counter is *E. coli* O157:H7. It's the pathogen that was responsible for the massive recalls of beef at Jack in the Box and Sizzler restaurants in California that spread to twenty-six states and made national headlines in 1993. (Now these types of outbreaks have become so commonplace that when they make the news, barely anyone notices.) Usually, this bug causes stomach cramps and diarrhea, but sometimes it can cause kidney failure and death. Children and the elderly are especially at risk.

But *E. coli* O157:H7 didn't become the problem it is today until we turned to the factory system of meat production, which consequently is now quickly being adopted by the rest of the world. Today, the average fast-food hamburger includes ground meat from dozens of states as well as from a few countries, like Argentina and Paraguay. This disease originates in the stomachs of cows and exits their bodies through feces. When cows stand in piles of their own excrement in massive feedlots, the pathogen then takes up residence in the bovine's urine- and feces-matted hide.

So when we're told to cook meat thoroughly to prevent foodborne illness, it's not because raw meat is inherently dangerous, but rather because cooking factory-produced meat thoroughly helps to kill off any dangerous bacteria that might be lurking in our hamburgers. No law requires slaughterhouses or industrial farms to test their facilities for the disease, and the USDA has no authority to demand a recall of tainted meat.

Don't despair: There are other choices. We'll get to them soon. But first, let's go take a look at the produce aisle. . . .

Mood Buster #4: MAD Vegetables

Meat's not the only thing that's changed. Step into the produce section of your favorite grocer and you're witnessing the most transformative aspect of grocery shopping: the cold chain. Thanks to a vast system of refrigerated warehouses, chilled tractor trailers, climate-controlled airplane cargo holds, insulated shipping containers, freezer holds, radio-frequency identification tags, and satellites, fresh lettuce can be harvested from California's Salinas Valley on a Monday and sold at a bodega in New York City's Lower East Side on a Wednesday.

The cold chain put an end to the idea of seasonality: Suddenly, anywhere in America, spring strawberries and summer tomatoes could be purchased in February. Except, of course, this bland, mealy produce tastes nothing like ripe, in-season crops. It's shipped from far-flung locales like Chile (the average piece of fruit travels 2,500 miles before you bite into it) and doctored so it looks more attractive (conventional oranges are injected with dye to brighten up their peels).

This produce is not cultivated for flavor but for how well it can withstand transport and storage without spoiling or bruising. The peach is a perfect example: Aficionados agree that nothing rivals the flavor of a ripe, just-picked peach, and that any type of refrigeration will lessen the taste. But ripe peaches are too delicate to survive the journey to a supermarket, so they're picked while they're still green. At best, the peaches you'll find at most grocery stores will be somewhat soft and palatable; at worst, they'll be shriveled and mealy.

Tomatoes are another example: They're picked immature and then, once they reach their destination, ripened artificially using ethylene gas. Shoppers often complain about the flavorless orbs, yet they continue to demand access to tomatoes year-round. As a result, scientists are scrambling to develop tomatoes that are both durable and better tasting. Massive energy-guzzling climate-controlled greenhouses, like the 318-acre Eurofresh Farms in southern Arizona, are springing up, and on test plots, new tomato varieties are being developed (the Tasti-Lee tomato, which took ten years to perfect, hit stores in 2010 and tastes nothing like an in-season variety).

All of this results in produce that's not nearly as healthy for us as it used to be. The crops that fill the cold chain grow year after year in the same fields and deplete soil of important trace minerals like magnesium that are crucial for brain health. Farmers then must make up for soil degradation by adding synthetic fertilizers derived from petroleum products to the fields. To ensure a good crop, fertilizers are usually overapplied. This makes plants "lazy" and means they don't have to produce as many nutrient antioxidants to defend themselves. Because the plants have such weak immune systems, farmers then need to spray them more heavily with pesticides. These are the vegetables that

THE STRANGE DOCTOR
WHO GOT AMERICA HOOKED ON PESTICIDES

Oil was discovered in Pennsylvania in the late 1800s, and at first the stuff was simply refined to make kerosene, a fuel that could be burned in lamps to light homes at night. Kerosene replaced candles made from animal fats and whale oil lamps because it was cheap and burned brighter. The only problem was that its production was messy and created a lot of waste that found its way into streams and rivers. These practices led to a lot of serious fish kills and spoiled waterways that livelihoods depended on. The refiners needed a use for the poisonous refuse. The solution, as it turned out, was right before their eyes. The deadly by-products of oil refining could be used to kill pests—bugs, rodents, birds. And thus pesticides were born. John D. Rockefeller's Standard Oil took the lead with a brand called Flit that was sold in hand-operated spray guns, a precursor to the modern-day aerosol can, to be sprayed in the home. To market Flit, the company hired a young illustrator named Theodor Seuss Geisel, who drew cartoons for the national humor magazine *Judge*. Geisel dreamed of one day becoming a writer, so he crafted a nom de plume to hide his identity while he worked on the ad campaign: Dr. Seuss. For the next seventeen years, he used his acerbic, over-the-top illustration style to advertise petroleum-derived pesticides. His catchphrase punch line, "Quick Henry, the Flit!" was as popular in the 1930s as Nike's "Just Do It" was in the '90s. Eventually, Theodor Seuss Geisel moved on to children's books, penning tittles like *Green Eggs and Ham* and *How the Grinch Stole Christmas!*

make up the produce section at the MAD grocery store. Fewer nutrients, more pesticides. Did we mention that they don't taste as good, either?

Nutrients Out, Toxins In

Of course, this approach to farming has serious drawbacks. Known as monoculture, growing one crop on a vast three-thousand-acre plot makes the plant an easy target for pests. Thus, massive amounts of pesticides are needed to grow the plants we MADly eat. Large monoculture crops deplete nutrients from soil, which explains why supermarket produce is about 40 percent lower in trace minerals than it was fifty years ago. The lack of these nutrients also makes the plants more susceptible to predators, and thus even more pesticides are needed.

We think of pesticides as chemicals that kill bugs, but in reality pesticides kill "pests." It's a blanket term that describes a whole host of chemicals that exterminate a wide range of pests, from fish to ferrets to fungi to fescue. Underneath the umbrella of pesticides are avicides (which kill pest birds), herbicides (which kill pest plants), and rodenticides (which kill pest mammals). Today in America, there are more than six hundred registered pesticides for use, and last year we applied more than 1.1 billion pounds of these chemicals on our crops, on our bodies, and in our homes.

The most widely used pesticide in the United States today is atrazine, which is applied to many of our most abundant crops, from cotton to soy. It interferes with hormonal signaling, and it's so powerful that repeated low-dose exposure turns male frogs into females—females that are fully capable of laying eggs. During the spring, atrazine concentrations in the water supply can hit one hundred times the EPA safety limit due to seasonal rains. Besides its impact on human health, the herbicide kills algae and grass along with disrupting reproduction of wildlife at the base of the food chain. Like a lot of other pesticides and chemicals still in use today in the United States, atrazine has been banned by the European Union. New research is beginning to prove some of our worst fears about this widely used pesticide, namely that it can disrupt our immune systems, impair insulin resistance, and promote obesity.

Researchers at St. Francis Hospital in Indiana recently described something known as the "June effect" in the Midwest: Children conceived in the early summer, after high doses of chemicals are sprayed on crops, are much more likely to have birth defects than those conceived at other times of the year.

TOP 100 REASONS TO AVOID PROCESSED FOODS

Even so-called sugar-free foods can still raise blood sugar—because they're sweetened with sugar alcohols like sorbitol, maltitol, and xylitol.

THE SECRET SCIENCE OF FOOD SYNERGY

Many of the dishes humans have eaten for generations—like rice and beans, or tomatoes drizzled with olive oil—have withstood the test of time not simply because the ingredients taste delicious together. Health experts believe we enjoy these combinations because they're more nutritious together than they are on their own. The concept is called "food synergy," and it explains how two foods can be greater than the sum of their parts. Here are a few of the most powerful food synergies currently known to science.

EGGS + CHEESE

The vitamin D found in egg yolks makes the calcium in dairy more available to your body—important not only for bones but heart health as well.

ROSEMARY + STEAK

Marinate your steak with rosemary before cooking: The herb is rich in antioxidants like rosmarinic acid and carnosic acid that help neutralize carcinogenic compounds known as heterocyclic amines (HCAs) that form when steak reaches temperatures of 325 degrees Fahrenheit or higher.

TOMATOES + OLIVE OIL

Cancer- and heart disease–fighting compounds called carotenoids (the most well known of which is lycopene) are found in abundance in tomatoes. They're fat-soluble and, as such, they're more available to your body when you eat them with fats like olive oil or mozzarella cheese.

GARLIC + FISH

Both of these foods fight inflammation and disease, but together, they're even more powerful: Research has shown that a combination of garlic and fish lowers LDL (bad) cholesterol more effectively than eating the foods on their own.

RASPBERRIES + CHOCOLATE

Scientists have discovered that when raspberries and chocolate are paired together, their disease-fighting flavonoids (quercetin in raspberries and catechin in chocolate) are even more effective at thinning the blood and improving heart health.

TURMERIC + BLACK PEPPER

The spice turmeric has anti-inflammatory properties—it's being studied for its potential to fight cancer, improve liver function, lower cholesterol, and stave off Alzheimer's disease. When you combine it with black pepper, your body absorbs a thousand times more curcumin (turmeric's active ingredient).

SALMON + RED WINE

Plant compounds in grapes known as polyphenols do more than promote good circulation—they also help your body absorb more of the brain-healthy omega-3s in fish.

OATMEAL + ORANGES

Phenols (a type of plant compound) in oatmeal and vitamin C in oranges both lower LDL (bad) cholesterol. When eaten together, their ability to improve cholesterol and prevent heart disease is four times greater than what they're capable of individually.

LEMON + SPINACH

The vitamin C in lemons helps your body absorb more of the plant-based iron found in spinach, a mineral that prevents mood swings and promotes happiness.

RED WINE + ALMONDS

Together, the antioxidant resveratrol in red wine and the vitamin E in almonds boost the body's ability to thin the blood and improve the health of blood vessel linings.

VINEGAR + SUSHI RICE

Vinegar decreases rice's ability to raise blood sugar levels by 20 to 40 percent.

BEET GREENS + CHICKPEAS

Chickpeas are a good source of vitamin B_6, which helps your body absorb the magnesium found in beet greens (B_6 helps facilitate the transport of magnesium across cell membranes). These nutrients work together in the body to ease the symptoms of PMS and ADHD.

GREEN TEA + LEMON

The vitamin C in lemon makes more of the catechins (a type of antioxidant) in green tea available to your body.

BANANA + YOGURT

Bananas contain inulin, which research indicates fuels the growth of yogurt's healthy bacteria (which helps regulate digestion and boost immunity).

APPLES + CRANBERRIES

These Thanksgiving staples are rich in a wide variety of antioxidants like quercetin and anthocyanidins; research shows that when you eat these foods together, their antioxidant activity is significantly higher than if you eat the foods separately.

THE SECRET SCIENCE OF FOOD SYNERGY—CONTINUED

CHICKEN + CARROTS

Chicken contains zinc, which is what your body needs to efficiently metabolize the beta-carotene in carrots into vitamin A, a nutrient you need for healthy skin, strong eyes, and a robust immune system.

FISH + BROCCOLI

Fish contains the mineral selenium, and broccoli is rich in a disease-fighting compound known as sulforaphane. Research shows that selenium and sulforaphane together are thirteen times more effective at slowing cancer cell growth than when eaten alone.

WHOLE GRAIN BREAD + PEANUT BUTTER

Together, these two foods contain all nine of the essential amino acids that your body needs to build bones, muscles, and hormones.

BROCCOLI + PINE NUTS

The vitamin C in broccoli helps keep the vitamin E in pine nuts active and potent.

BLUEBERRIES + WALNUTS

Blueberries contain phytochemicals known as anthocyanins that protect the brain from oxidative damage, and walnuts are a rich source of omega-3s that make you smarter. Research has shown that these compounds are even more powerful at sharpening memory and improving communication between brain cells when they work together.

GARLIC + ONIONS

The organosulfur compounds in garlic and onions are more powerful in combination than alone. Together, they help remove plaque from arteries and keep blood vessels flexible and healthy.

Many of our most widely used pesticides are known as persistent organic pollutants (POPs). That means that they don't break down easily in the environment, and they accumulate in our bodies and food. DDT is the most infamous POP, and our government banned it in 1972 after, among other things, it nearly killed off our national symbol of freedom, the bald eagle. A 2010 study in Dallas of 310 food items found that DDT's main metabolite, DDE, is the most prevalent and concentrated pesticide found in food. POPs like DDT are fat-soluble, which means that they accumulate in fatty tissues—like those that make up the human brain.

Preschool children who eat conventionally raised food have six times as many pesticide metabolites compared to those who eat organically raised food. Today, pesticides taint one-fifth of the average American child's daily food.

Aside from contributing to acute toxicity and lower IQs, chronic low-grade exposure to pesticides leads to disrupted metabolism and neuropsychiatric disorders like depression, Parkinson's, and Alzheimer's disease. Beyond these chemicals' neurotoxic and carcinogenic effects, a study of 33,457 licensed pesticide applicators demonstrated that pesticide exposure increased their risk of diabetes by up to 94 percent. No matter how you slice it, your food is much better off without these man-made toxins.

A MAD Synergy

When you add multiple chemicals together, there is often a synergistic effect, meaning the whole is greater than the sum of its parts. For example, smokers exposed to asbestos are much more likely to develop lung cancer.

Unfortunately, we can't yet predict how the sixty-seven different pesticides found on celery interact with one another and affect our health, though a study of coho salmon published in 2009 in *Environmental Health Perspectives* sheds some light on the issue. Researchers found that individual exposure to five of the most common pesticides had no effect on salmon, but certain combinations of those same chemicals were deadly. More often than not, the application of pesticides is done without regard to any potentially toxic interaction.

Scared yet?

That's not really our intention. We want to get you riled up enough to make a change that will ultimately make you happy and healthy. It's that simple. You can be happier. You can be healthier. And now we're going to show you how.

Next up: the good news.

4

Good Food, Good Mood

When humans hunted and gathered their food, they ate a much wider variety of plants. Evidence appears in the stomach contents of what are known as "bog men," early Europeans who thousands of years ago fell into—or were discarded in—peat bogs, where their bodies were mummified. One of the most pristinely preserved of these humans, known as Grauballe Man, came from modern-day Holland and foraged during the Iron Age. His stomach was stuffed with sixty-six different species of plants—an astonishing variety considering today we only eat about twenty different plants and that this sample described only what Grauballe Man had for his last few meals. We also know that this diversity was not unique. Aboriginal Australians ate 150 different kinds of roots and some three hundred different types of fruits. In the New World, Native Americans ate a vast variety of vegetables, including corn (yellow, blue, red, white, black . . .), squash (spaghetti, Hubbard, pumpkin, fairytale pumpkin, buttercup . . .), beans (black, pinto, climbing, green . . .), chile peppers (Aji, hatch, paprika, habanero, serrano . . .), and many varieties of edible plants. Thomas Jefferson grew more than 150 species of fruit and some 330 vegetables on his estate, Monticello, in Charlottesville, Virginia.

The vast majority of medicines were discovered in plants. These chemicals make up the plant's defenses, the plant's immune system. Since plants are immobile, they have to protect themselves by creating poisons that make them unappetizing to predators. That's why plants have antibacterial properties inside your gut. But it's more than that; plants, like humans, also have to defend themselves against other dangers like heat waves and intense sunlight. Many do so with the compound lycopene, found in summer fruits like tomatoes and watermelon. Eating these fruits also boosts your skin's ability to cope with the sun.

Plants must also protect themselves from oxidative stress, which, in humans, leads to inflammation, something that is emerging as an underlying cause of brain disorders like depression and Alzheimer's disease as well as heart disease and cancer. Many plant compounds (phytonutrients) travel to the brain, where they fight inflammation and activate genes that boost our innate antioxidant defenses. Others promote the formation of new brain connections and the birth of new brain cells.

Plants contain minerals, vitamins, and phytonutrients that have been used for decades to boost and stabilize mood. As the science of phytonutrients evolve, the mechanisms by which they improve cognition and memory are increasingly discovered.

Plants improve blood flow to the brain and protect its blood supply. Certain phytonutrients, like quercetin, actually enter arterial plaques and help break them up, reducing the risk of dementia, heart attack, and stroke. Phytonutrients block compounds that cause cancer and trigger precancerous cells to self-destruct. They boost our liver's ability to eliminate toxins in the blood. Studies show that when plants are exposed to

TOP 100 REASONS TO AVOID PROCESSED FOODS

The pigments that make grapes purple and pumpkins orange protect brain cells, while the artificial ingredients that mimic these colors in processed foods can impair brain function.

32

TOP 100 REASONS TO AVOID PROCESSED FOODS

Kraft Stove Top Stuffing contains propyl gallate, a substance that was recently discovered to interfere with the hormone estrogen, which regulates sexual desire and mood in women.

stress, like a brief drought or attacks by a swarm of aphids, they have a threefold increase in the concentration of beneficial phytochemicals like polyphenols, a major family of plant compounds responsible for many of the brain-building and inflammation-fighting actions of plants.

We've coevolved with plants in ways that are sometimes surprising, but as we've replaced the foods we've been eating for thousands of years with sugar, refined carbohydrates, and industrial-toxin-filled foods, we've forgone an amazing bounty of nutrients that are responsible not only for promoting health but also for our happiness.

We call these "lost" nutrients the Essential Elements of Happiness. As you'll see, these nutrients tend to travel together—gangs we want on our side—to fight low mood, low energy, cloudy thinking, as well as all the diseases associated with the metabolic syndrome. That means not only do these elements promote happiness, they also keep you trim and strong.

They're found in some places you might expect, like the plants we've been discussing, specifically leafy greens, and others you might not, like butter and lard.

Let's take a look at each of the nutrients that make up the Essentials:

1.	Vitamin B_{12}	7.	Fiber
2.	Iodine	8.	Folate
3.	Magnesium	9.	Vitamin A
4.	Cholesterol	10.	Omega-3s
5.	Vitamin D	11.	Vitamin E
6.	Calcium	12.	Iron

Essential Element of Happiness #1: Vitamin B_{12}

No nutrient makes a better argument for eating animal products than B_{12}. You can't make brain cells without this vitamin. Low B_{12} causes irritability, depression, and cognitive decline. Certain bacteria that live in the guts of animals are the only organisms that make B_{12}. As such, these animals accumulate the nutrient in their tissues, and you'll find high concentrations in cows, goats, and other ruminant animals and in seafood such as fish and shellfish. Our stomachs make a special protein called intrinsic factor to absorb B_{12} from our food. B_{12} also regulates the expression of genes, meaning it prevents things like cancer from happening.

Thanks to a host of factors related to modern life, it's difficult to get enough of this essential element into our bodies. People who are especially at risk of deficiency are those who have digestive problems, especially acid reflux, celiac disease, and irritable bowel syndrome. Alcohol also leaches B_{12} from the body. Another problem is that most processed foods are fortified with folic acid, which masks B_{12} deficiency, additional signs of which are aggression, obsessive-compulsive behavior, sleeplessness, and tingling in the arms and legs.

Long-term effects of B_{12} deficiency include heart disease, cancer, and Alzheimer's. It is estimated that up to 40 percent of women and of the elderly have suboptimal levels of B_{12}. Vegans and vegetarians, of course, are at risk of deficiency. While the ethical decision of not eating meat is laudable, it's important to realize what that means nutritionally, and many plant eaters who return to animal products report a big boost in mood that is likely related to B_{12}.

A Healthy, Happy Dose

If you have symptoms of B_{12} deficiency or a condition that might lead to deficiency, ask your doctor to check your B_{12} levels. Don't settle for low levels even if they are "low normal." Two hundred to 1,100 picograms per milliliter is normal, but levels of under 400 increase your risk of mental health problems like dementia and depression. It's important to note that supplementation of this vitamin—like vitamin E, folic acid, and others— has been linked to an increased rate of cancer and death. Therefore, if you're suffering a deficiency from malabsorption (which can often be attributed to common drugs, like antacids), try to get to the bottom of the underlying problem rather than treat it with a supplement. Most antacids, for example, block this Essential Element.

BEST SOURCES: Shellfish, fish, liver, beef, eggs.

Essential Element of Happiness #2: Iodine

If ever there was a nutritional case to be made that life originated in the ocean, iodine is evidence of it. Iodine is a nutrient that all animals need for life, and it can be obtained only through diet. Iodine is essential for a healthy thyroid—the gland that regulates metabolism. An underactive thyroid is associated with low energy, poor memory, depression, ADHD, migraine, weight gain, infertility, breast disease (including cancer), infection, and heart disease.

Proper brain development requires iodine; in fact, iodine deficiency is the most common cause of preventable brain damage in the world. Iodine is a rare mineral in nature, and it's mostly found in the ocean because, like salt, it dissolves in seawater. The highest amounts of this nutrient are found in seaweed, and scientists speculate that's why Japanese women have a much lower incidence of breast cancer than women in the United States.

Convenience foods are wreaking havoc on bodies' ability to use iodine. Soybeans can be processed into everything from candles to industrial solvents to biodiesel, but most of it ends up in our food. While soy has been hyped as a health food, it's loaded with compounds known as goitrogens, substances that block iodine absorption by the thyroid. Typically, the salt added to cheap convenience foods is not iodized, because iodized salt is more expensive. These foods also often contain potassium bromate, which is added to baked goods as a dough conditioner. This chemical has been banned in almost every country because it causes cancer (especially in the breast). Virtually the only place it's still allowed to be used is in the United States. Processors like the additive because it's widely available and cheap. The problem is that it's structurally similar to iodine and blocks this Essential Element from being absorbed by the thyroid.

Aside from baked goods, potassium bromate is added to some pumpkin seeds, like those sold by Planters. Citrus sodas like Mountain Dew contain a similar additive called brominated vegetable oil. Bromine, the father element, is used in the popular pesticide methyl bromide, which is sprayed on tomatoes, strawberries, and processed meats. It's being phased out because it destroys the ozone, but the United States has sought numerous exemptions—such as California's strawberry crops.

If all of that weren't enough, our homes are swimming in a sea of brominated flame retardants. They're put in our clothes, furniture, and electronics to prevent house fires. These chemicals have been banned in Europe, and they're increasingly being linked to health problems the more they're studied. When it comes to avoiding bromines in your home, look for labels like "flame retardant free" or "PDBE-free."

Since the 1970s, the iodine levels in Americans have dropped in half. There are a handful of reasons for this, but one result is a lot of unhappiness. When you don't get enough of iodine, you're much more likely to suffer mood disorders. Women need more iodine than men because breasts use a lot of iodine, and scientists now believe that's why women who don't get enough of this nutrient often have lumpy chest tissue (fibrocystic breasts) and experience extra breast pain during menstruation.

A Healthy, Happy Dose

While seafood is one of the richest sources of iodine, seaweed contains hundreds of times more iodine than fish.

BEST SOURCES: Seaweed, fish, clams, shrimp, sardines, eggs, grass-fed meat and milk, potato skin.

Essential Element of Happiness #3: Magnesium

Magnesium is a mineral that eases your mind, nerves, and muscles. It's even been used to treat clinical depression. It protects your brain from the waste product ammonia, relaxes blood vessels, and protects against heart disease and diabetes. Increasing magnesium levels in the brain improves memory and learning, while a deficiency can lead to depression, anxiety, ADHD, insomnia, and fatigue.

The USDA estimates that one-third of Americans are deficient in magnesium, while other government surveys report that almost 70 percent of us don't eat enough of this vital nutrient. Industrial farming is stripping our soil of this mineral, and the majority of our calories—refined carbs, vegetable oils, and sugar—are devoid of magnesium. Some prescription medications for high blood pressure, like the diuretics Lasix and hydrochlorothiazide, increase magnesium loss from the body, as does having high blood sugar.

A Healthy, Happy Dose

Plants use magnesium to make the green pigment called chlorophyll, which is what they use to convert sunlight into energy. To get enough of this natural antidepressant, you need to eat greens—foods such as spinach, beet greens, collard greens, broccoli, green beans, and Swiss chard.

TOP 100 REASONS TO AVOID PROCESSED FOODS

Zinc is known as the "the intelligent mineral," and it's removed from grains when most manufacturers make processed foods.

Whole grains are also high in magnesium, as are fish like halibut and wild Alaskan salmon. One of the best sources of magnesium, however, is a sugar that used to be abundant in our diet: molasses. Use it in place of table sugar in everything from coffee to baked goods.

BEST SOURCES: Green leaves, whole grains, salmon, beans, sunflower seeds, blackstrap molasses.

Essential Element of Happiness #4: Cholesterol

Cholesterol is not the dietary demon that it's been made out to be. While you've heard a lot about this substance and its role in heart disease, you've probably *not* been told that its highest concentrations are found in your brain. Another top source of this amazing nutrient? Breast milk.

There are two points we want to hammer home. First, eating cholesterol in your diet has a very small impact on your blood cholesterol levels. Second, avoiding high cholesterol foods, like eggs and salmon, means you're missing out on some of the richest sources of essential brain nutrients.

Cholesterol is a waxy substance found in the cell membranes of all animals. In the brain, it forms a protective layer around your neurons and facilitates the near-hypersonic transmission of nerve signals. The brain makes cholesterol locally, which is perhaps why some studies have suggested a link between statin medications (those that block cholesterol synthesis) and low mood. While the science is just emerging, we know that chronic cholesterol depletion disrupts neurotransmitters that regulate mood. Low cholesterol levels have been linked to an increased risk of suicide and are also associated with an increased risk of cancer.

Not only are your brain cells made from this nutrient but so, too, are your hormones, the chemical messengers that regulate your body's most basic tasks. Cholesterol plays a crucial role in the formation of bile acids that allow our bodies to break down dietary fat and absorb the fat-soluble vitamins A, D, E, and K.

The reason we were originally misled about this amazing nutrient is that when doctors in the 1950s looked at the new epidemic of heart disease, they noticed that most patients had one thing in common: deposits of plaques. Scientists analyzed the material and found that it contained, among other things, cholesterol, a substance barely understood at the time. (Note that a main ingredient in arterial plaque is calcium—yet no one is rushing in to blame calcium for heart disease.) Experts knew that cholesterol accounted for a significant portion of our brain's weight and that it was manufactured by our livers, but apart from that they didn't know much else.

In 1961, *Time* magazine profiled Ancel Keys, America's most famous proponent of the saturated fat/cholesterol theory of heart disease, which proposed that saturated fats elevate blood cholesterol and the prevalence of heart disease. Keys was a physiologist from the University of Minnesota who had developed the army's rations for World War II—the K ration. Keys simplified the story of cholesterol before it was studied or fully understood. "A remarkable substance apart from its tendency to be deposited in the walls of arteries," he told the magazine. The *Time* story strongly advised Americans to limit their consumption of butter, milk, and eggs because they contained cholesterol, and confusion about dietary cholesterol and its influence on blood cholesterol persists today. But from this reasoning was born the idea of nutrient-deficient foods—fat-free milk, margarine, and egg whites—as health foods.

Getting a Clearer Picture

We've learned a lot since the 1960s. Dietary cholesterol is not the "bad" guy. It's a more complicated picture than what Keys painted. To further explain, let's take a look at the oft-maligned but ever-edible egg.

Aside from a human's first dietary staple, breast milk, no other food is as cholesterol-rich as egg yolks. It's no coincidence; both eggs and milk are filled with nutrients that are important for growing brains, hearts, and bodies. Today, we know that pasture-raised eggs are also a good

TOP 100 REASONS TO AVOID PROCESSED FOODS

The first ingredient in Kraft Light Creamy French bottled dressing is high fructose corn syrup.

34

source of omega-3s—a protective fat for our brains and hearts that wasn't even discovered until the 1970s.

Eggs, like breast milk, are loaded with B vitamins, which are important for gene expression. They also contain the nutrient choline, which lowers blood levels of homocysteine, a marker of cardiovascular disease and depression.

Three of the highest egg-consuming nations—Spain, France, and Japan—have the lowest rates of cardiovascular disease. As a result, Harvard University decided to put the old theory that eggs raise our blood cholesterol to the test. They gathered 115,000 nurses and physicians to report egg consumption, and after fourteen years the results were clear. Eggs don't raise blood cholesterol in those who eat up to seven a week (it's hard to find people who eat more than that) and don't raise the risk of heart disease, stroke, or death. They actually appear to have *protective* roles against the disease we were told they cause.

It's true that the cholesterol tests that your doctor runs are predictors of heart disease, *but what's wrong is the explanation of how diet causes your cholesterol to become out of whack.* Your body contains about one hundred grams of cholesterol, nearly all of which is produced by your liver. At any given time, around 10 percent of this amount is coursing through your veins. An egg, again one of the richest cholesterol sources, contains about 135 milligrams of cholesterol—that's less than 1 percent of the amount of cholesterol already being pumped around your body. For the majority of Americans, eating foods high in cholesterol doesn't raise blood cholesterol substantially. Think of it this way: It's impossible to eat enough cholesterol to supply your body's needs—that's why it's manufactured by the liver.

Instead, a diet high in sugar, refined carbohydrates, and vegetable fats—the MAD—is what causes plaques to form in the arteries. These foods spike blood sugar, which your body turns into triglyceride fats to deposit around your waist. It's this process that leads to obesity, diabetes, and atherosclerosis. But don't take our word for it; Walter Willett, MD, the head of nutrition at the Harvard School of Public Health, has been sounding the alarm about refined carbs and heart disease for the better part of a decade.

It's time to cut out the refined carbs and industrial vegetable fats. That means avoiding the oils from corn, cottonseed, safflower, sunflower, and soy. They were created and marketed to be a safe alternative to animal fats high in cholesterol. Millions of people dutifully made the switch. Then fifty years later, scientists made an alarming discovery: These new hydrogenated fats were high in trans fats. They double heart disease risk and greatly increase the risk of getting depressed. Now, food processors are racing to remove them from all the most popular processed foods—crackers, cookies, ice cream, chips, and, yes, margarine. A review published in *The New England Journal of Medicine* went so far as to deem these fats the worst macronutrient in existence for heart health. Yet healthy eaters had been consuming them for decades to lower their risk of this very disease.

A Healthy, Happy Dose

Don't be afraid of high-cholesterol foods like butter, whole milk, eggs, and fatty fish. There's a reason we've been eating these foods for millennia. If you have cholesterol numbers that put you at risk for heart disease, try lowering them by eating the Happiness Diet. After all, sugar, carbohydrates, and trans fats found in the MAD are what's most clearly linked to heart disease.

With so much emphasis on lowering cholesterol, you might be surprised to hear that high levels of cholesterol have been linked to *better*

TOP 100 REASONS TO AVOID PROCESSED FOODS

Fructose, a sweetener found in most processed foods, blocks leptin, a hormone that tells your brain you are full.

memory and mood in healthy middle-aged and elderly people. Perhaps even more surprising, though, is to learn that as people get older, higher levels of total cholesterol are associated with a decreased risk of dementia, according to researchers from Johns Hopkins University Bloomberg School of Public Health. And not only that, but researchers at the Danish Aging Research Center at the University of Southern Denmark have found that those over age eighty with high cholesterol have a decreased risk of death from all causes.

BEST SOURCES: Eggs, salmon, meat, milk, cheese, lard from sustainably raised pigs.

Essential Element of Happiness #5: Vitamin D

There's a reason why the sun feels so good on our skin—just like plants, we need it for survival. Sunshine converts cholesterol in our skin into vitamin D, an essential nutrient that controls the expression of some two thousand genes. (Is it any wonder so many cultures have worshipped the sun?) Low levels of vitamin D are linked to a host of mental disorders, including depression, dementia, Parkinson's disease, premenstrual dysphoric disorder, and seventeen types of cancer. Vitamin D deficiency is also linked to lowered immunity. Some researchers now believe that one reason we get sick in the winter months is because we get less sun exposure—and therefore less vitamin D. Many people now believe that this lack of vitamin D is a culprit behind seasonal affective disorder. A low vitamin D level increases both the risk of getting depressed and the severity of depression in the elderly.

For decades, doctors have mainly focused on vitamin D's role in bone strength, as it is needed to absorb calcium from our digestive system into

TOP 100 REASONS TO AVOID PROCESSED FOODS

The FDA allows nineteen maggots and seventy-four mites in a three-and-a-half-ounce can of mushrooms.

cells that "mineralize" our bones. Osteoporosis (weakening of the bones) affects more than 55 percent of the population above the age of fifty. To fix this problem, public health officials have focused on increasing our consumption of calcium. But without vitamin D, we absorb less than 10 percent of the calcium in our diet.

Vitamin D is fat-soluble. That means we actually need fat in our diet to absorb this essential nutrient. We're not the only animals that rely on the power of vitamin D for life—far from it. That means some animal foods—like salmon and chicken eggs—are full of this nutrient.

People spend much less time in the sun today than they used to, and when they do go outdoors, they're likely to be slathered in sunscreen from head to toe. Sadly, sunscreens block 99 percent of the UVB rays our skin need to produce vitamin D. Our daily commutes also play a role. Before the automobile, we were all exposed to many more UVB rays. Glass blocks this wavelength of light, so if you're in a car, train, or bus, you're not getting hit with them. Our cities are more polluted than they used to be, and particulate matter—you guessed it—also blocks sunlight from activating our vitamin D stores. Not only that, but many people live in cities crammed with tall buildings that further obstruct sunlight.

Many doctors now recommend a supplement to make up for this deficiency. Recently, the Institute of Medicine increased its daily recommendation for intake of vitamin D from 400 IU to 600 IU. However, many health experts believe that even 600 IU is woefully inadequate. Left to its own devices, our skin can produce more than 10,000 IU of vitamin D in just thirty minutes. We don't recommend supplements for the most part, but during the wintertime, we do make an exception for vitamin D.

People who have darker skin are much more likely to be vitamin D deficient. It's because skin tones developed to match populations' level of sun exposure. Traditionally, humans who lived near the equator had darker skin to protect them from intense, year-round sun. People with lighter skin lived in more northerly climates, where their fair complexion evolved to help them make *more* vitamin D during the short daylight of the winter months. But now we're free to live wherever we want, and as more people with dark skin move to more northerly climates, like those of the United States and Europe, more people are likely to be deficient in this nutrient. Today, 90 percent of Americans with pigmented skin (African American, Hispanic, and Asian) have insufficient levels of vitamin D.

Another risk factor for vitamin D deficiency is . . . being born in contemporary America. Newborns are completely dependent on breast milk or formula for all their nutritional needs, and the amount of vitamin D in breast milk is dependent on a mother's vitamin D status. Unfortunately for fetuses and newborns, more than half of pregnant women have low levels of vitamin D. Studies show that the lower the vitamin D level in a mother's blood at the time of birth, the lower the birth weight of the child (which is linked to all kinds of problems from learning disorders to a lower income later in life).

Not only has our relationship with the sun changed, but as we've stated repeatedly, so, too, has our food. We used to eat voraciously from the food chain's offering of vitamin D–rich foods: seafood and pasture-raised animal products. Yet never before have such large populations lived so far from the ocean. Consequently, we eat much less fish. We gave up another very important source of dietary vitamin D: lard. Before America

---

TOP 100 REASONS TO AVOID PROCESSED FOODS

A massive recall of Kroger-branded frozen vegetables happened because the company believed the products might contain glass fragments.

was inundated with cheap industrial vegetable oils, we cooked with pig fat at every meal—and as you've learned, this essential vitamin is fat-soluble. When sows spend their lives rooting around outdoors, they are exposed to massive doses of sunlight, making lard an excellent source of this nutrient. Imagine that: Before science knew vitamin D existed, our great-grandparents were eating it all winter long.

A Healthy, Happy Dose

Make sure your vitamin D level gets checked during your annual doctor visit. Experts recommend getting fifteen minutes of direct sun exposure daily, or a few thirty-minute sessions a week. If that's too difficult during the short days of winter, talk to your doctor about taking a supplement, and make sure it's labeled as D_3. Odds are you'll be happier and a lot healthier. It's important to eat fatty fish like salmon, tuna, and sardines, which are top sources of this Essential Element of Happiness. So, too, is pasture-raised lard, which you should rotate into your cooking repertoire.

BEST SOURCES: Sunlight, fatty fish, butter and lard from pasture-raised animals, mushrooms (must be exposed to the sun).

Essential Element of Happiness #6: Calcium

You probably think of calcium as important when it comes to bone health, but calcium also regulates the electrical circuitry of our brains and hearts. Calcium triggers the release of neurotransmitters into the synapse every time a neuron fires. This element mediates the internal response of a neuron when receptors on the surface of the cell are stimulated. Calcium is involved in the survival of neurons and the formations of new connections by regulating the expression of the genes that make BDNF.

Disturbances in calcium levels can produce anxiety, depression, irritability, impaired memory, and slow thinking. When calcium levels are low in your bloodstream, the nutrient is leached from your bones to make up for the inadequacy, which is what leads to osteoporosis. A constant deficiency creates a hormonal imbalance that causes weight gain and women to suffer severe PMS symptoms.

The majority of Americans don't get enough calcium in their diet. While doctors used to think this deficiency was because we didn't eat enough of this nutrient, it turns out that's not the whole story.

America's calcium problem likely has to do with the fact that we're chronically deficient in its cofactor, vitamin D. Insufficient vitamin D means we can't process calcium. Making matters more complicated, calcium supplementation has been linked with illnesses like heart disease and cancer.

A Healthy, Happy Dose

The top dietary sources of calcium are dairy products like yogurt, milk, and cheese. If you need to avoid dairy, great options are leafy greens (that's why grass-eaters like cows are able to build the strong bones necessary to support their weight). Note that some leafy greens, like spinach, contain oxalic acid, which interferes with calcium absorption but is easily neutralized by cooking. Our favorite source of calcium? Sardines. Consumption of this fish replete with its small bones provides a robust serving.

BEST SOURCES: Sardines; milk; yogurt; cheese; kale; cabbage; collard, mustard, and turnip greens; spinach; almonds, pecans, and walnuts.

TOP 100 REASONS TO AVOID PROCESSED FOODS

Candy corn is actually made with corn—corn syrup.

Essential Element of Happiness #7: Fiber

Think of fiber as the conductor of the complex orchestra that is your digestive system. Extracting all the nutrients your brain needs takes a healthy gut.

Diets low in fiber have been linked to depression and increased risk of suicide. One reason is that fiber is an indicator you are eating foods like whole grains and plants that contain the other Essential Elements of Happiness. Another is that fiber reduces overall inflammation. Fiber helps you avoid spikes in blood sugar and insulin, which over time cause a deterioration of the blood-brain barrier that keeps toxins out of the brain, so they can't disrupt mood regulation, memory, and brain growth.

Before modern food processing, everyone ate a diet high in fiber. But nowadays, many of us are fiber deficient because the manufacturing process strips fiber from the food because it's too expensive to keep it intact during processing and it's cheaper to add it back later. Today, food manufacturers add unnatural fiber sources such as bamboo to processed foods. These new forms of fiber are reported to give people diarrhea, bloating, and allergic reactions. They can also block absorption of key nutrients like iron, calcium, and zinc.

A Healthy, Happy Dose

Boosting the fiber in your diet is as easy as following one simple rule: Eat more plants. Don't rely on processed foods with fancy food claims for this Essential Element.

BEST SOURCES: Green leafy vegetables, cruciferous plants like cauliflower and broccoli, beans, fruit.

Essential Element of Happiness #8: Folate

Folate keeps your neurotransmitter factories humming. The cerebospinal fluid that bathes your brain has four times more folate than does your blood. Higher concentrations of folate in the blood are linked to a decrease in negative mood states, clinical depression, and fuzzy thinking. Folic acid has been used for decades to treat clinical depression. Folate also improves mood by boosting the production of the long-chain omega-3s DHA and EPA, helping create compounds like defensin-1 that protect the brain from inflammation.

Folates increase concentrations of acetylcholine in the brain, the neurotransmitter that disappears in memory disorders like Alzheimer's disease. More folate in your diet improves memory and cognition. Folate also keeps homocysteine levels low, which decreases your risk of low mood and promotes better functioning of your arteries, protecting your brain from a stroke. In fact, Big Pharma recently took notice of the importance of folate in mental health and started marketing a prescription version of this plant metabolite called Deplin. The FDA requires food processors to add synthetic folic acid to processed carbohydrates. While we know that natural folate promotes mental health and protects against heart disease and cancer, there is major concern about the synthetic version of folate (folate acid), which has been linked to cancer and asthma. Synthetic folate also masks symptoms of B_{12} deficiency, which is widespread and can lead to irreversible cognitive decline if not diagnosed early.

Scientists haven't yet determined why folic acid is less effective than naturally occurring folate, but it may have something to do with the fact that in nature, folate is found in eight different forms. In other words, in the plants you eat there are eight totally unique (though chemically similar) folates. The synthetic version comes in only one form and may be too simple for the complexities of gene expression.

A Healthy, Happy Dose

Folate is very sensitive to heat and light. To maximize its content in food, choose fresh leafy greens—kale, Swiss chard, Boston lettuce, beet greens—and eat them raw or cook them lightly. That means steam instead of boil. Choosing locally grown greens decreases the amount of time from harvest to table and increases folate content.

If you're on a budget, keep in mind that freezing foods doesn't damage this Essential Element of Happiness. Your frozen-food section is a great resource when the plants you like to eat are not in season.

BEST SOURCES: Spinach, kale, black beans, black-eyed peas, lentils.

Essential Element of Happiness #9: Vitamin A

If you've heard about vitamin A, it's likely because someone told you that carrots have a lot of this nutrient and that it's good for your eyes. Carrots are high in compounds called carotenoids that can be converted into vitamin A, but this process can be very inefficient. The only place vitamin A is found in its usable form is in animal fats. That's why sailors have long depended on cod liver oil for night vision—not carrots.

The area of our brain that's responsible for giving birth to new brain cells, the hippocampus, is loaded with receptors for vitamin A. This nutrient plays a powerful role in the expression of DNA in neurons. Specifically, it promotes the production of the enzymes that make neurotransmitters like dopamine and their receptors, the key players in the basic biochemistry of mood, memory, and learning.

What you might be surprised to learn, though, is that the most important source of this nutrient is meat.

Our misguided obsession with low-fat foods means many of us have stopped eating great sources of vitamin A: egg yolks, liver, whole milk, and butter. We've largely replaced these foods with fats that are totally deficient in vitamin A. While taking a supplement sounds like an easy fix, the synthetic form of this nutrient has been linked to lung cancer. Large doses of synthetic vitamin A from supplements can cause serious birth defects, and the acne medicine Accutane, a synthetic form of vitamin A known as 13-cis-retinoic acid, has an FDA warning for depression and suicidal thoughts.

A Healthy, Happy Dose

The best source of vitamin A is chicken, pig, or beef liver. Your body is very efficient at storing this nutrient, so that means eating pâté (or a similar dish made of liver) a few times a month is more than enough to make sure your brain has the vitamin A it needs to produce new brain cells.

BEST SOURCES: Liver, egg yolks, shellfish, butter, and whole milk.

Essential Element of Happiness #10: Omega-3s

Omega-3s are a group of essential fatty acids required by every cell in the human body. These special fats came to the attention of scientists in the 1970s when they noticed that populations of Eskimos who ate a high-fat diet had no heart disease. Diets high in omega-3s are known to prevent depression, obesity, cancer, heart disease, and many, many other ailments. Omega-3s are popularly associated with fish, but most people don't know that they actually originate in the leaves of plants. The reason they're so high in fish is because the bottom of the oceanic food chain is phytoplankton—microscopic leaves.

There are actually three types of omega-3s. The first type is the form found in plants, known as alpha-linolenic acid (ALA). Animals convert this fatty acid into two higher forms known as eicosapentaenoic acid (EPA) and docosahexaenoic acid (DHA). These are the two forms that we use in our brain and in our hearts. These two fats are metabolically active, meaning nature uses them to do some of the most amazing things.

Humans use them to form complex thoughts and build hearts that can beat billions of times without stopping. Salmon use them to migrate thousands of miles through cold ocean waters. These fats are also found in the tail of sperm and the wings of hummingbirds. If you want to think fast or run quickly, you want a diet rich in these crucial fats.

Before omega-3s were discovered to be essential to brain and heart health, food processors removed them from their products because they spoil easily, preventing manufactured foods from having a long shelf life. Also, the animals we ate, prior to current livestock-raising practices, were high in omega-3s because they spent their lives foraging on grass and grass-eating grubs.

A Healthy, Happy Dose

Humans do a terrible job converting ALA into the higher forms of EPA and DHA. That means flaxseed oil is no match for fish oil. While fish oil supplements will certainly help you meet your daily needs, we recommend eating fish instead because there are so many other important nutrients found in it that are essential to happiness, like B_{12}, zinc, and iodine. After all, the long-living populations of places like Japan don't survive on fish oil but on fish.

Other good sources of omega-3s include grass-fed milk, butter, cheese, pasture-raised beef, chicken, eggs, and pork. It's important to remember that these fats are in constant competition with omega-6s for space in our cells. This means eating more omega-6s found mainly in processed food makes it harder for your body to reap the benefits of brain-building omega-3s.

Increasingly, naturally raised meats are being sold in gourmet grocers around the country. To find out more about where to find these foods, see Chapter 8, "Shopping and Stocking Your Kitchen."

BEST SOURCES: Fatty fish like sardines, mackerel and salmon, free-range eggs, and grass-fed meat.

TOP 100 REASONS TO AVOID PROCESSED FOODS

Eight ounces of macaroni is permitted to contain 225 insect fragments and 4.5 rodent hairs.

Essential Element of Happiness #11: Vitamin E (Tocopherols and Tocotrienols)

Vitamin E is a generic catchall term that describes a family of eight anti-oxidants known as tocopherols (alpha, beta, gamma, and delta) and tocotrienols (alpha, beta, gamma, and delta) that protect fat. Vitamin E protects the fats in our brain from free radicals, especially the omega-3 fats DHA and EPA, which are concentrated in neurons. Emerging science shows tocotrienols are important neuron protectants, as they block inflammatory signals that kill brain cells. In studies of the elderly, those who eat a variety of tocopherols from food show a significant decrease in both cognitive decline and the onset of Alzheimer's disease. And patients with clinical depression have significantly lower vitamin E levels. Aside from protecting your neurons, natural forms of vitamin E are also linked to the prevention of cancer and protection from heart disease. *Synthetic* alpha-tocopherol has been linked to cancer and heart disease, while the complex arrangement of natural forms prevent these diseases.

A Healthy, Happy Dose

According to the USDA Center on Human Nutrition and Aging at Tufts University, less than 10 percent of us get adequate levels of vitamin E. Processed food and supplement manufacturers rely on just one form, alpha-tocopherol; we make sure you get all eight.

BEST SOURCES: Almonds, olives, beet greens, turnip greens, collard greens, and Swiss chard.

Essential Element of Happiness #12: Iron

The areas of the brain with the largest concentrations of iron are those related to memory, learning, and mood. It is a vital cofactor in the synthesis of the mood-regulating neurotransmitters dopamine and serotonin.

Iron is needed for brain cells to produce energy and is particularly important for proper brain development. Teenagers with low iron levels perform worse on cognitive tests, and infants with iron deficiency have learning and concentration problems later in life. As the center of the protein hemoglobin, iron is our body's basis for transporting oxygen. All this iron makes your blood red—just like the red planet Mars. Iron also is the core of important proteins in the body that form the cytochrome system in our liver that rids our body of toxins. Detox diets that promote fasting or juice? Foods high in iron—like shellfish and beef— are a better bet.

Insufficient iron intake is the number-one nutritional deficiency in the United States. With nutrition claims on cereal boxes that boast "100 percent of your daily iron needs," you may wonder how it's possible that this deficiency is so widespread. There are two forms of iron in our food: nonheme iron found in plants, and heme iron found in meat. We can only absorb small amounts of the plant iron, while we absorb up to 35 percent of the animal iron.

A Healthy, Happy Dose

Don't rely on fortified foods for your iron needs. The best source of iron is shellfish—clams have more than ten times the amount of iron as beef. Also keep in mind that your body needs acid to best absorb iron, which

THE HEALTHY SUGARS

Recently there's been a lot of debate (and much misinformation) about the health hazards of high fructose corn syrup. While it's true that HFCS is bad for your health, that's not because it's different from table sugar. The problem with HFCS is that it's found everywhere in the Modern American Diet, so we're eating way too much of the stuff. Heavily processed sweeteners—like white table sugar and HCFS—have no nutritional value. But we didn't always fill up on these nutritionally void sweets. Until rather recently, we primarily used natural sweeteners that contained beneficial vitamins and minerals. Here's a look at a few:

HONEY

Honey contains essential B vitamins, folate, iron, manganese, and fluoride. It contains 181 different bioactive compounds such as the polyphenol antioxidants quercetin and caffeic acid that boost energy production in the brain, prevent cancers from forming, and fight inflammation. It also helps to fight seasonal allergies and has strong antimicrobial properties (it's even been shown to kill the antibiotic-resistant superbug MRSA). The FDA has gone so far as to approve honey-dressing bandages for infections.

MAPLE SYRUP

Long before Europeans arrived on American shores, Native Americans tapped hardwoods like beech and maple to make *sinzibuckwud,* a syrup that translates to "drawn from wood." Pure maple syrup contains minerals such as manganese, zinc, calcium, iron, and antioxidants. But we mean *real* maple syrup. What you generally encounter in the grocery store is a mix of HFCS and caramel-colored dye. Maple syrup has a thinner consistency and has a unique mix of flavors based on the time of year, the temperature during the time of harvest, and the mix of nutrients in the soil. Many of the subtle flavors of maple syrup represent flavonoid compounds that have reported antitumor and antioxidant qualities, such as vanillin, coniferol, catechin, and coumaric acid. A serving of maple syrup contains about the same antioxidant capacity as a serving of strawberries.

BLACKSTRAP MOLASSES

Molasses was the most popular sweetener in the United States until the 1880s. Refined sugar is made by boiling the juice from sugar cane or sugar beets and then bleaching the extracted crystals. Molasses is the leftover liquid after the raw dark sugar crystals are removed. Molasses contains vitamin B_6, magnesium, manganese, iron, calcium, copper, and selenium. A tablespoon of molasses has as much iron as a chicken breast.

means antiacid medications could be zapping your iron levels. Supplements such as calcium, zinc, magnesium, and copper are also known to block iron absorption. Why not get these nutrients in their natural form anyway?

BEST SOURCES: Shellfish, grass-fed beef, duck, dark chicken meat, and liver.

Part 2

The Happiness Diet:
The Foods, Menu Plans, and Recipes

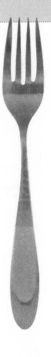

5

Food for Thought

Every cell is made up of fats. The human brain is 60 percent fat. And many vitamins essential for brain function, like A, D, E, and K, are fat-soluble. Your body cannot absorb these nutrients without fats. So the idea that we should be stripping fats from our diet is absurd. We should instead be searching out the best fats possible, especially if we want our brains to function sharply, smoothly, and efficiently—the subject of this chapter. What are the best foods for enhancing mental function? We'll zoom in on five of our favorites, our Focus Foods, and explain why you should eat them if you want a sharper, sounder mind. Of course, as with all of the Happiness Diet foods, these have crossover benefits that overlap with our recommendations for good mood foods and energy-boosting foods. Sometimes we couldn't choose just one, so we give you a couple or even a "group"—as in the case of our number 1,

TOP 100 REASONS TO AVOID PROCESSED FOODS

A University of Cincinnati study found that a diet high in fructose and trans fat doesn't just lead to obesity—it also causes oxidative damage to the liver that decreases your body's ability to eliminate toxins.

which is a three-way tie: eggs, grass-fed beef, and dairy. A good rule of thumb to remember is that when it comes to whole foods, the greater the variety, the more sharp, merry, and energized will be your mind.

Top Five Focus Foods
1. Eggs, grass-fed beef, and milk
2. Brussels sprouts
3. Grapefruit and lemon
4. Berries
5. Anchovies

Focus Food #1:
Free-Range Eggs, Grass-Fed Beef, and Milk

Eggs

What if we could create the perfect brain food—one that could fix the problems in the MAD way of life? What would it look like? Let's pretend for a minute and imagine this magical food.

For starters, we'd want to load it up with B vitamins, since those have been stripped from refined carbohydrates. Let's begin with B_6, since it's crucial for most all of your cognitive functions. Next, we'd toss in some B_{12}, the vitamin that is so important that true vegetarians often need to take a supplement. B_{12} is crucial for avoiding agitation and loss of focus. Together, these two vitamins would do a lot to lift fatigue across America. They'd also go a long way toward boosting memory and treating nervousness and depression.

Next we'd add B_9, also known as folate. Not only will this nutrient protect your brain, but it will lower homocysteine levels in the blood (high levels are one of the best predictors of cognitive decline). B_9 will also protect our DNA from damage, something that leads to the genesis of cancerous tumors.

TOP 100 REASONS TO AVOID PROCESSED FOODS

Little Debbie gingerbread cookies contain titanium dioxide, a white dye
found in paint that damages DNA and is listed as a possible human
carcinogen by the International Agency for Research on Cancer.

It'd make sense as well to toss in another Essential Element of Happiness: iodine, the element that is central to our metabolism's master switch, the thyroid.

We should next add the trace minerals that have been stripped from America's soil by the monoculture crops of corn, soy, and sorghum. So let's add magnesium, since it's the mineral that will loosen up our muscles and relax our circulatory systems, helping us focus on the tasks at hand of daily life. Next up is zinc, a mineral that improves brain function and helps B_9 regulate our gene expression so that we stay healthy. We should add iron to this wonder food, too. This trace metal will boost our body's ability to transport oxygen around our bloodstream and further increase energy and focus.

Since we have all of these B vitamins and iron, let's add a complete protein with lots of tryptophan so that we will have all the basic ingredients for the most important mood-regulating neurotransmitters like serotonin, norepinephrine, and dopamine.

Now, even though it's not found in many foods, let's get creative and add some vitamin D. It's something most of us are deficient in, as we've changed our relationship with the sun. Clearing up this deficiency will severely lower more than a dozen of the most deadly cancers, among many other ailments.

Let's see, what else? How about some cholesterol? Yes, that's a great idea, since that's what your body uses to manufacture vitamin D from the sun—so we'll be working twofold to clear up this deficiency. Cholesterol is also crucial because it's a main component of bile, which is what your gut will use to absorb this amazing amount of nutrients we're combining to make this miracle food.

Lastly, let's throw in some omega-3s, since we all know these fats make us smarter and protect us from heart disease. Wait . . . one more thing. For good measure, let's have Mother Nature design this food. We know she works in mysterious ways that we often subvert when we try to outsmart her genius.

You've just read the nutritional profile of a standard barnyard egg—a nutritional powerhouse that's created by nature when a hen lives a normal life foraging around a farm.

Beef and Dairy

We've been bombarded with the terms *polyunsaturated, monounsaturated,* and *saturated.* We're told to eat olive oil because it's high in "good" monounsaturated fats and not to eat butter because it's high in "bad" saturated fats. While trans fats from hydrogenated vegetable oils are certainly the most deadly things to come around since cigarettes, this obsession over good fat and bad fat is lot of nonsense. And nowhere is this more true than with beef and dairy, which contains conjugated linoleic acid, or CLA—a fat you need to know more about.

Fat is not the enemy.

What the marketers don't tell us is that the fats in our food are a mixture of polyunsaturated, monounsaturated, and saturated. Recently, scientists at the University of California, San Diego School of Medicine decided to profile human blood and map the different fats found within. They found 588 different types of fat.

"For the first time, we've identified and measured hundreds more and ultimately we might discover thousands," Edward A. Dennis, PhD, of UC San Diego told *Medical News Today.* "These numbers and their remarkable diversity illustrate that lipids have key, specific functions, most of which we do not recognize or understand."

But we do know some generalities: We do know that eating sustainably and naturally raised meat and dairy fights depression, builds brain cells, and trims your waistline—among other things. CLA is the only fat recognized by the US National Academy of Sciences to inhibit the growth of tumors. It's only found in meat and animal products (milk, cheese, yogurt, butter, cream), specifically grass-fed ruminants.

CLA increases blood flow to the brain, protects brain cells from death caused by hyperstimulation (called excitotoxicity), and counteracts the effects of the stress hormone cortisol. Grass-fed animals have 300 to 500 percent more CLA than grain-fed ruminants.

The most concentrated sources are found in milk and cheese, especially from sheep and goats; and the meat of beef, lamb, goat, and bison. CLA prevents some cancers, promotes muscle growth, and prevents abdominal fat deposits. Researchers call CLA a body composition modulator, as it reduces body fat (especially around the waist) while increasing muscle mass.

When you consider that a human's first food is milk from our mothers' breasts, it's not surprising that humans have been milking ruminant animals like goats, sheep, and cows for thousands of years. Today, though, there's a lot of confusion about dairy and whether or not it's something that humans are "supposed" to eat. Some populations never developed the trait that enables humans to break down the sugar in milk known as lactose throughout adulthood (the majority of the world's people lose this ability around the age of five). Many cultures around the globe, including much of the Asian world, are lactose intolerant and

TOP 100 REASONS TO AVOID PROCESSED FOODS

Most processed foods contain at least one—if not several— soy-derived ingredient. While considered to be healthy, consumption of soy products is associated with cognitive decline and brain atrophy.

have stomachs that can't handle dairy because they've never needed to and got their nutrients elsewhere—like, in the case of the Japanese, from the sea.

The United States is full of people of Northern European descent (many artisanal cheeses originate in countries like Switzerland, Spain, and France) who do have this ability. Our species developed the ability to digest lactose several times throughout the history of humanity because milk, butter, yogurt, and cheese are such nutritious—and by our ancestor's standards, convenient—foods. Before refrigeration, a goat or a dairy cow meant an endless supply of perishable food, one that carried itself down the trail on its own four legs. Dairy—along with seafood—is one of the few dietary sources of iodine, a mineral essential to the regulations of metabolism. Concentrated dairy products like yogurt and cheese contain higher levels of iodine than milk. Unlike plants, dairy is a complete protein source that contains all of the amino acids your body needs to build and maintain things like brain tissue, eyes, organs, muscles, and even the collagen that keeps your skin tight and wrinkle free. And just like beef, dairy is an excellent source of CLA, that amazing fat that actually promotes weight loss around the belly.

A quick glance at the nutrients in pasture-raised butter turns up a laundry list of beneficial nutrients: phosphorus, potassium, magnesium, selenium, fluoride, calcium, folate, choline, betaine, vitamin B_5, vitamin D, vitamin K, omega-3s, and CLA.

The consumption of dairy is linked to a reduced risk of heart disease, stroke, and diabetes, along with an increase in good HDL cholesterol and

TOP 100 REASONS TO AVOID PROCESSED FOODS

The preservative disodium dihydrogen pyrophosphate, found in things like Ore-Ida Tater Tots and "all natural" Alexia Roasted Red Potatoes & Harvest Vegetables, is also used as an oil dispersant.

lower blood pressure. Now that you've heard so much about the amazing benefits of CLA, we'd like to introduce to a few other fats that play all kinds of roles in optimum brain functioning and overall health.

Eating Meat Is Good for the Brain?

Yes. Meat is brain food. By picking the right meats you get a food source packed with brain nutrients and not empty calories. Meat from seafood is the most concentrated source of the long-chain omega-3 fatty acids EPA and DHA. These fats are needed to make healthy brain cells and to promote the synthesis of BDNF, a molecular Miracle-Gro for the brain.

Meat contains heme iron, which is the most highly absorbable form. The brain is dependent on a constant flow of oxygen, and this process depends on eating enough iron (red meat is red because it has a high iron content). Meat is the most concentrated form of vitamin B_{12}—people with lower B_{12} levels lose more brain volume as they age—and the best source of zinc. Zinc consumption can improve academic performance, which means smarter kids. Meat also triggers hormones like leptin that let your brain know when you are full.

Meat is a great source of brain-essential nutrients, but some of you have reasons to avoid meat. While you can get all of your nutrients from meatless sources using supplements, it is a much more complicated endeavor.

Focus Food #2: Brussels Sprouts

As omnivores, humans are designed to eat from a much wider variety of foods than simply animal products. Variety is the spice of life, as they say, and it's what keeps your brain running on all cylinders. So next up is a vegetable from a group of plants that have been shown to have some pretty extraordinary brain-boosting benefits: crucifers.

HAPPY FATS/MAD FATS

HAPPY FATS

ALPHA-LINOLENIC ACID (ALA)

WHY YOU NEED IT: Used to produce other omega-3s vital to brain function. Linked to a reduced risk of depression.

Find it in flaxseed, purslane, walnuts, kale, brussels sprouts, pasture-raised meat, and eggs.

EICOSAPENTAENOIC ACID (EPA)

WHY YOU NEED IT: Cools inflammation in the brain, thins your blood, and relaxes blood vessels. Reduces your risk of brain disorders like depression and dementia.

Find it in seafood, especially fatty fish like salmon and mackerel, shellfish, and grass-fed beef, bison, and lamb.

DOCOSAHEXAENOIC ACID (DHA)

WHY YOU NEED IT: The top omega-3 in your brain, it is vital for healthy connections and the production of molecules like neuroprotectins and resolvins that protect brain cells. Low levels are linked to a host of brain disorders ranging from ADHD to suicidal thoughts.

Find it in sardines, salmon, anchovies, and (for vegetarians) certain types of algae.

CONJUGATED LINOLEIC ACID (CLA)

WHY YOU NEED IT: Counteracts stress hormones, decreases belly fat, and increases blood flow to the brain.

Find it in the meat, milk, and cheese from pasture-raised ruminants (beef, lamb, goats).

OLEIC ACID

WHY YOU NEED IT: Used to make memory-boosting oleoylethanolamide and linked to a decreased risk of depression and diabetes.

Find it in almonds, olive oil, lard, beef, and most fish.

CAPRYLIC ACID

WHY YOU NEED IT: Helps new brain cells grow, fights inflammation, and helps regulate hunger.

Find it in coconut and palm oil, milk, and cheese.

STEARIC ACID

WHY YOU NEED IT: Boosts innate brain cell antioxidants and is essential for healthy memory and mood function.

Find it in chocolate, meat, and dairy.

NERVONIC ACID

WHY YOU NEED IT: Found in brain cell insulation (myelin) and decreases your risk of obesity and heart disease.

Find it in flaxseed, hemp seeds, salmon, mustard, and human breast milk.

MAD FATS

LINOLEIC ACID

WHY YOU *DON'T* NEED IT: This omega-6 fat promotes inflammation and is linked to increased risk of depression and diabetes. While essential, there is a vast excess in the MAD.

Find it in vegetable oils like corn, soy, cottonseed, safflower, and sunflower oils and factory-farmed meat.

ELAIDIC ACID

WHY YOU *DON'T* NEED IT: The major trans fat in the MAD clearly linked to heart disease and depression.

Find it in partially hydrogenated vegetable oils.

INTERESTERIFIED FAT

WHY YOU *DON'T* NEED IT: Industrially produced unnatural saturated fat designed to replace trans fats. These are completely new to the human diet and appear to interfere with sugar processing and cholesterol levels.

Find it in many processed foods listed as "high sterate" or "steric rich" or with "interesterified" fats.

TOP 100 REASONS TO AVOID PROCESSED FOODS

When you buy processed foods, you help fund the ten billion dollars spent every year to market junk foods to kids. Since 1980, obesity has tripled among adolescents.

The thousands of phytonutrients found in cruciferous plants are so complex that science is truly only starting to understand them. What we do know, however, is that these compounds evolved over millions of years to help plants fight disease and attack from predators. It makes sense that these nutrients would be beneficial for us as well. These are things like the complicated-sounding indole-3-carbinol, which is being studied by the National Cancer Institute for its ability to stave of the nation's number-two killer. Our body converts this molecule into diindolymethane, also known as DIM, which activates our immune system to kill viruses and bacteria. Nothing "dim" about that.

DIM can also stop cancer cells from forming and spreading. Nothing *dim* about that. Brussels sprouts protect your brain with the phytonutrient sulforaphane, which guards new brain cells sprouting in our hippocampus . . . even as we age.

Focus Food #3: Grapefruit and Lemon

Another powerful family of plants is citrus. All citrus—grapefruit, oranges, limes, lemons, tangerines, and so on—are closely related and can interbreed. They're said to be promiscuous that way, which explains why new varietals like the tangelo, a tangerine-grapefruit hybrid, continue to pop up.

TOP 100 REASONS TO AVOID PROCESSED FOODS

The production of soy—an ingredient used in cookies, crackers, breads, and many other packaged foods—is the largest cause of deforestation in Brazil.

TOP 100 REASONS TO AVOID PROCESSED FOODS

Atrazine, a popular herbicide, contaminates much of America's waterways.

Botanically speaking, all citrus are actually berries, because each fruit comes from a single ovary. In fact, nearly every fruit—from the banana to the avocado—is a berry. Citrus originated in China and have been cultivated for at least 2,500 years. That's why in Puerto Rico the word for orange is *china*. Citrus fruits are known for their high levels of vitamin C, which was important for fighting scurvy when sailors spent long times at sea without access to fresh greens. Scurvy is not a concern today for modern humans, but diseases from a diet of excess are, and citrus appear to protect against those, too.

Citrus fruits contain many members of the flavonoid family of phytonutrients, like hesperetin and naringenin, that are able to cross the blood-brain barrier. While flavonoids are often touted for their antioxidant capacity, these molecules don't seem to simply eliminate free radicals. Once in the brain, flavonoids reduce inflammation, eliminate neurotoxins, repair damaged neurons, and promote the formation of new connections between neurons. Flavonoids also enhance mental functioning by improving blood flow to the brain. This is why the Happiness Diet menus and recipes are rich with these compounds.

Naringenin, the flavonoid responsible for the bitterness in grapefruit juice, blocks the enzyme acetylcholinesterase, just like modern medicines that treat Alzheimer's disease. It also decreases LDL cholesterol, improves insulin sensitivity, and is being investigated for the treatment of diabetes and obesity. And it's a key reason why we've chosen grapefruit as one of our Focus Foods.

Hesperetin protects neurons from dying during a heart attack or stroke. It also protects neurons by recharging antioxidants like vitamin C and increasing amounts of the powerful antioxidant superoxide dismutase (SOD) in the brain.

TOP 100 REASONS TO AVOID PROCESSED FOODS

Blue No. 2, a dye originally used in textiles but now found in M&M's and other candies and desserts, is linked to brain cancer.

And if you feel that citrus soothes you, it might be because hesperetin also binds to our opioid receptors, the same target as heroin and Oxycontin. Another compound in citrus, tangeretin, a flavonol found in tangerines, protects the nigrostriatal neurons from toxins, the same neurons that die off in Parkinson's disease.

Citrus fruits are focus foods because they're loaded with limonoids, a set of phytochemicals that keep your brain cells healthy by maintaining their antioxidant systems. Limonoids have proven anticancer activity as well, stopping the growth of breast and brain cancer. They increase the activity of certain chemotherapeutic agents tenfold and prevent the formation of lung, skin, colon, and oral cancers in laboratory animals. Limonoids are known to induce the production of glutathione in our liver, a substance known as the "master antioxidant," enhancing its ability to remove carcinogens from our blood.

Certain limonoids have even been shown to inhibit the replication of the HIV virus. Others signal our liver to produce less LDL cholesterol, which is linked to heart disease. So far scientists have discovered over three hundred limonoids—molecules you'll never find in a vitamin C pill or a multivitamin.

Limonoids are most concentrated in the skin of citrus, which makes sense because that's the fruit's first line of defense against pests. That means you should own a zester so that you can shave off a little lemon, orange, or lime atop your morning yogurt or into sauces and soups for extra flavor and protection against heart disease and cancer.

Just be sure you zest only organic skins, because this is also the part of the citrus berry where pesticides—many of which are neurotoxic—accumulate.

Focus Food #4: Berries

Now let's turn our attention to those fruits that are often thought of as brain food: berries. You're about to be thrown a botanical curveball because those fruits—blueberries, strawberries, and raspberries—aren't technically berries at all. Berries are defined as fruits that come from a single ovary, like a grape. Strawberries are actually what are known as accessory fruits, because their seeds are on the outside. Raspberries and blackberries are aggregate fruits, which means that each little fleshy bulb of fruit on those "berries" comes from its own ovary. The reason these

IN PRAISE OF THE PUMPKIN

The biggest berries are found in the plant family Cucurbitaceae, which is made up of all the world's squash and melons. That means everything from a cucumber to a watermelon to the record-holding 1,725-pound pumpkin grown by Christy Harp of Jackson Township, Ohio, are all berries—most so big that the only thing strong enough to bear their weight is terra firma.

Most of the pumpkin we eat comes in cans from Morton, Illinois, where Nestlé turns the state's harvest into Libby's brand. That's a shame, because canned pumpkin doesn't even play a close second fiddle to fresh roasted pumpkin, the taste of which Hernando de Soto likened to the flavor of chestnuts all the way back in 1539. Pilgrims used to slice this squash's top off, scrape out the seeds, and fill the pumpkin with apples, molasses, spices, and milk. They baked the concoction whole. Early Americans also used to brew pumpkin beer, a tradition that is being revived by boutique breweries like Dogfish Head. Italians roast pumpkin and cover it with shavings of Parmigiano-Reggiano and aged balsamic vinegar. Pumpkin, one of the thousands of squash varieties, has been eaten for hundreds of years to ease bladder problems, to dampen symptoms of PMS, and to boost vision. The latter use makes sense, because pumpkin is high in beta-carotene as well as a molecule known as beta-cryptoxanthin that significantly lowers your risk of lung cancer.

Pumpkin extract is now in clinical trials to treat diabetes, because this fruit appears to make the pancreas grow back after it's been damaged by too many years of MAD. Pumpkin seeds—like all squash seeds—are packed with the amino acid tryptophan that our brain uses to make neurotransmitters like serotonin. Pumpkin seeds have even been shown to reduce social anxiety.

"berries" are a little grainy is because you eat the seed within each of these bulbs. Why is that important? Because these seeds contain the highest amount of the phytochemicals known as ellagitannins that rid our bodies of neurotoxins like pesticides and plasticizers.

When it comes to protecting your brain, think deep reds and purples. Raspberries, blueberries, Concord grapes, plums, eggplants, and red cabbage get their color from a set of compounds called anthocyanins that protect the neurons at the center of our brains responsible for feeling and memory.

Remember to eat a mix of different berries to reap the full array of brain benefits. In animal studies, blueberries were shown to improve spatial memory by increasing the amount of brain-health promoting BDNF in the hippocampus, a key brain area for memory, while strawberries are loaded with fisetin that can improve long-term memory (and decrease the complications of diabetes). The take-home point is clear—berries are a top concentrated source of powerful phytonutrients that cross the blood-brain barrier. Once in your brain, these molecules turn on genes that cool inflammation and promote new brain connections and growth.

And last but not least, cranberries contain a unique phytochemical called proanthocyanidin that prevents bacteria from adhering to the bladder. That's why it prevents urinary tract infections.

Focus Food #5: Anchovies

You might associate this fish with pizza, but there's much more you can do with it, and it's easy to prepare in a way that even the kids will eat.

TOP 100 REASONS TO AVOID PROCESSED FOODS

Low-fat, highly processed dairy products get stripped of conjugated linoleic acid (CLA), a fat that fights cancer and prevents abdominal fat deposits.

Anchovies have ten times as many omega-3s as tuna. Kids who get more of these fatty acids have higher IQs. These fish are healthier than tuna for another reason: They're so low on the food chain, they're often free of contaminants like mercury and persistent organic pollutants like DDT.

If you wonder how it's possible to get these fish in your diet in way that's tasty, it's really simple. Make a savory dressing out of them to top any of the Happiness Diet vegetables (see page 218).

In addition to their brain-boosting abilities, the omega-3s in anchovies can reduce your risk of a heart attack by 50 percent, decrease triglycerides, and improve HDL, the good cholesterol. Anchovies are packed with vitamin D, which is essential for fighting off the blues and building bones. They're loaded with coenzyme Q10, an essential molecule that has been shown to slow down the progression of Parkinson's disease and improve cardiovascular function. Anchovies are also a top dietary source of calcium.

The Happiness Diet Brain-Sharpening Foods

Almonds	Coconut milk	Mussels
Blueberries	and oil	Onions
Brussels sprouts	Garlic	Pears
Butter	Grapefruit	Pumpkin seeds
Clams	Lard	Walnuts

6

Food for Energy

Eating for energy is a little trickier than eating for mood or brainpower. That's because exercise plays a role in what you can and can't eat. Put simply: If you're an endurance athlete, your body is constantly cycling through your food, and you can afford to eat more carbohydrates because they'll quickly be burned off.

For most of us, that's not the case, and we should avoid plants that are easily assimilated by our bodies and converted into sugar: aka simple starches. Are these foods inherently bad for you? No. At least when eaten in moderation. But will these simple starches make you fat and shrink your brain if you eat too many of them? Yes. They'll also spike and crash your blood sugar, leaving you with little to no energy. This is the problem with the MAD way of eating.

51 TOP 100 REASONS TO AVOID PROCESSED FOODS

A McDonald's Happy Meal purchased by Sally Davies, a New York–based artist, showed no signs of decomposition after *six months*.

People eat cereal or a bagel for breakfast with some orange juice, and then by 11:30 their energy has crashed and they're craving lunch to get them going again. At lunch, they'll eat some pasta or perhaps a submarine sandwich, and the process starts over again. Blood sugar spikes and then falls again, leaving them with cravings in the afternoon.

Instead, we'd all do better to focus on complex carbohydrates that are broken down into sugar and enter the bloodstream at a regulated pace, maintaining energy. These plant foods keep your digestive system running smoothly and make sure your gut absorbs nutrients effectively. The best choices for complex carbohydrates are high-fiber foods such as leafy greens like beet greens, mustard greens, and turnip greens; lettuces; cabbage; broccoli; asparagus; and cauliflower. You'll also get slow-burning complex carbs in whole grains like barley and brown rice and legumes such as beans and chickpeas. But those aren't the only plants you should be consuming for more energy. What are our favorites? Here you go:

Top Five Energy Foods

1. Mesclun
2. Drupes—coffee and chocolate
3. Walnuts
4. Red beans
5. Blue- or red-skinned small potatoes

TOP 100 REASONS TO AVOID PROCESSED FOODS

Kellogg's brand assorted fruit snacks that come in shapes inspired by Disney movies like *Finding Nemo* and *Toy Story 3*, contain carnauba wax, a substance commonly used in car wax and shoe polish.

Energy Food #1: Mesclun

An important nutrient that originates in the leaves of plants is vitamin B_9, also known as folate, which you've heard us talking about quite a bit already. Its name comes from the Latin word *folium*, for leaf. This nutrient protects our bodies from depression, heart disease, and cancer. That's because folate works as a methylator of DNA. That's a science-y word that essentially means this nutrient makes sure your genes are expressed correctly as you grow older. Or, to put it another way: Without folate, biological processes go out of whack and we get sick. Researchers have noted that many cancerous cells have low levels of methylation. And mothers who are folate deficient are more likely to give birth to babies with neural tube defects.

But leaves contain so much more than folate, which explains why humans have been eating salads for thousands of years. One of today's most popular lettuces, *Lactuca sativa* L., is believed to have been first cultivated on the Greek island of Kos, and that's why today many cultures know it as "cos." The Romans passed the leaf onto the French in the 1300s, who gave it the name you are more likely to know it by: romaine.

While it's much more nutritious than iceberg, romaine comes in behind our top pick: mesclun.

The best way to reap the benefits of eating leaves is to consume as wide a variety as possible—as each species has its own set of phytonutrients. A good start is the mesclun mix at the grocery store. Two leaves usually found in this assortment—beet greens and oak leaf lettuces, for

TOP 100 REASONS TO AVOID PROCESSED FOODS

People who eat foods with artificial sweeteners often end up consuming more total calories per day. It's likely because these sweeteners are so much sweeter than sugar that they prime the brain's desire for even more sweet foods.

TOP 100 REASONS TO AVOID PROCESSED FOODS

Azodicarbonamide is used to manufacture plastics and foam. While banned as a food additive in the European Union and linked to developing asthma, you'll find it in Wonder Bread and Stroehmann Dutch County 100 percent whole wheat bread.

example—mean a hefty dose of red pigments called carotenoids, which boost levels of the superdetox molecule in our liver, glutathione, and reduce the oxidation of cholesterol that leads to arterial plaques.

Leaves are the most nutrient-dense food we eat. One cup of arugula has just twenty-five calories but contains most of your daily need for folate, vitamin K, vitamin C, calcium, fiber, and beta-carotene.

As a kid, you probably remember being told a thousand times what a great source of calcium milk is, but you probably weren't told that leaves are also packed with calcium. Generally speaking, the darker the leaf, the better. That deep green comes from the Essential Element of Happiness known as magnesium, which eases our nerves, relaxes our blood vessels, and protects us from heart disease. Plants use magnesium to make chlorophyll, the green substance that converts sunlight into energy. So the more exposed a leaf is to light, the more magnesium it will contain, which is why the outside leaves are always darker than those on the inside.

Many of the most nutritious greens need to be cooked because they either have tough textures or they're bitter and sautéing mellows them. These are leaves like kale and mustard greens, and they're superconcentrated with spicy, sulfur-containing antioxidants that stave off mental decline, heart disease, and cancer. These are also crucifers (the family includes brussels sprouts, bok choy, collard greens, and cabbage). Heating them turbocharges their sulforaphane content, a compound that literally kills precancerous and cancerous cells. Sulforaphanes ignite the liver's detoxification system, sweeping out toxins before they damage your body and brain.

Energy Food #2:
Drupes—Coffee and Chocolate

Coffee

Coffee is the extract of the coffee drupe, which is a type of fleshy fruit that surrounds a hard shell with a seed inside. Drinking this morning staple is proven to improve memory and reflexes.

Methylxanthine is the phytonutrient commonly known as caffeine. In the brain it blocks the action of a neurotransmitter called adenosine, which inhibits the firing of other neurons, particularly dopamine and glutamate neurons. By releasing the adenosine "brake," coffee causes a boost in mental activity, focus, and mood. Dopamine and glutamate activity increase in an area of the brain called the nucleus accumbens; this area modulates pleasure and influences focus and decision making via connections to the frontal lobes.

Other stimulants like amphetamine and cocaine influence the same brain area, and while coffee is not as powerful or addictive as these drugs, people become irritable and get a headache if they suddenly stop drinking coffee. In addition to its stimulating properties, a cup of coffee has more antioxidant phytonutrients than a glass of grape juice or a serving of spinach. Scientists believe this is why it can protect your liver from the damage of drinking alcohol and reduces inflammation throughout the body.

Some of these terms are brain teasers in and of themselves, but these compounds and substances are crucial to powering your brain (and hey, brain teasers are good for keeping you sharp, too!).

Coffee contains two beta-carboline phytonutrients, norharman and harman, that function in the brain like the class of drugs called monoamine

TOP 100 REASONS TO AVOID PROCESSED FOODS

Drinking too much soy milk may lower a man's sperm count.

TOP 100 REASONS TO AVOID PROCESSED FOODS

Legally, 6 percent of potato chips is permitted to contain some rot.

56

oxidase inhibitors that are used to treat depression and Parkinson's. These compounds are likely contributors to the association between those who drink a few cups of coffee daily and a decreased risk of brain disorders.

A study in Finland followed 1,409 people for an average of twenty-one years and found that those who drank three to five cups of coffee daily had a 65 percent reduction in the risk of developing dementia. Coffee is also linked to a reduction in the risk of diabetes and heart disease. A massive study published in the *Archives of Internal Medicine* (it covered 457,922 people) found that for each cup of coffee consumed, people had a 7 percent reduction in the risk for diabetes. But of course, as we all know, you can overdo it on coffee, too. And that's why we recommend rotating coffee with other stimulating, phytonutrient-rich beverages, like green and black tea, and limiting yourself to a few servings a day. Remember, drinking these beverages late in the day can disrupt sleep.

Chocolate

This brings us to perhaps the most lusted-after fruit on the planet: cacao—also known as chocolate. While cacao is the Aztec name for this drupe, Carl Linnaeus, the Swedish botanist who created the nomenclature we use to categorize all living things, gave it another name: *theobroma*, food of the gods. We couldn't agree more.

Chocolate is loaded with flavonols like epicatechin that improve blood flow to the brain, reduce neuron damage after stroke, and protect against dementia. A recent study from the *Journal of Psychopharmacology* shows that a few ounces of dark chocolate a day improves mood (maybe you already knew this?) and increases brain processing speed—all the while reducing mental fatigue.

Consuming a small amount of dark chocolate daily protects your heart by lowering blood pressure and blood sugar. It even makes cells more sensitive to insulin, improving their ability to process sugar. Chocolate contains phytonutrients that increase energy expenditure and protect against weight gain. It also reduces levels of the stress hormone cortisol. Just don't forget: the darker the chocolate, the better.

Energy Food #3: Walnuts

The strategy of the fleshy fruit is to attract animals' attention with bright colors and sweet sugars so that their seeds are carried off and deposited where they can continue the gene pool. There's a second type of fruit, however, that has a different strategy for spreading its seed.

These are known as dry fruits, and their flesh shrivels up into a tough shell to protect the plant's seed until it's ready to sprout. Most of the world's calories come from the dry fruits of soy, corn, wheat, and rice. (Bet you didn't know these were fruits.) We commonly know these dry fruits as seeds or grains.

And just like the skin of fleshy fruits, the skin of dry fruits is nutrient dense. When you hear that it's healthy to eat "whole grains," that's because you're eating the skin of the "grain"—technically known as bran. This is stripped away during processing to prolong the shelf life of processed foods. Along with the bran, the germ is stripped out during processing. Together these two parts contain 90 percent of the dry fruit's phytonutrients that are so complex we don't yet have the science to understand all of their benefits. The germ of whole grains is a lot like an egg yolk, and it's where the DNA and many nutrients are held for the next generation. This is why nutritionists like to say junk food is full of empty calories—it's been stripped of these nutrients.

Some seeds are so big we call them by another name: nuts. And one of our favorites, for so many reasons, is the walnut.

Stop and think for just a second how amazing a walnut is. You can fit one in the palm of your hand—yet it has all the building blocks to grow into a tree as wide as a school bus and as tall as a ten-story skyscraper.

Nuts, like eggs, were demonized during the 1980s and 1990s because they're fatty. Now we understand that those fats aren't unhealthy and that both eggs and nuts are loaded with trace minerals and vitamins like magnesium, copper, iron, manganese, zinc, calcium, omega-3s, vitamin E, folate, B vitamins—sort of like a multivitamin, except designed by nature. Additionally, walnuts have a 1 to 3 ratio of omega-3s to omega-6s that humans thrived on until the rise of industrial fats.

We also now know that the fats in nuts actually help us absorb many of the other nutrients within this seed. Vitamin E, for example, is fat-soluble and comes in eight different forms in nature. The various forms of vitamin E work to cool off brain inflammation and protect neurons, which may explain why patients with depression often have low levels of vitamin E in their blood. In addition to acting as antioxidants that guard the fats in our brain, the different forms of vitamin E prevent inflammation by regulating genes that express inflammatory factors.

Nuts are high in fiber, a nutrient that is associated with a decreased risk of heart disease, diabetes, and obesity. A study of 31,208 Seventh-day

TOP 100 REASONS TO AVOID PROCESSED FOODS

58

Salmonella found in Jennie-O turkey burgers that prompted a recall of 55,000 pounds of meat in April 2011 was resistant to the most commonly prescribed antibiotics.

Adventists found that those who consumed nuts at least four times a week were 48 percent less likely to die of a heart attack.

Energy Food #4: Red Beans

Another type of seed is the legume, which we know more popularly by two different names: beans and peas.

These seeds are laid in pods and have been staple foods for thousands of years. That's because they're a great source of protein—not to mention fiber, magnesium, folate, and iron. There are dozens of varieties of legumes: black beans, snap peas, black beans, red beans, adzuki, navy beans, and on and on the list goes.

The USDA tested the antioxidant capacity of 147 of the most commonly eaten plant foods. On the top of their list (and ours, too) were red beans, with an antioxidant capacity of 13,727, closely followed by red kidney beans, with 13,259. Red beans have 65 percent more antioxidant power than the oft-touted miracle fruit: the blueberry. (We're not picking on berries here; you know we love them. But we do want to make you aware that marketing and science don't often tell the same stories.)

Both red and black beans are high in anthocyanins—the same compounds found in most berries—which contribute to their health-promoting reputation. Data are accumulating to show that these compounds influence gene expression in the brain in ways that improve communication between cells and protect neurons from the effects of aging.

Just remember to soak your beans overnight; soaking releases the seeds' phytates, which will otherwise block your body's ability to absorb

TOP 100 REASONS TO AVOID PROCESSED FOODS

The FDA allows 5 percent of any jar of maraschino cherries to contain maggots.

some important nutrients like magnesium and calcium. (Thankfully, soaking tampers down the gassy side effect of eating beans as well.) Snow peas and green beans are totally fine to eat raw.

Energy Food #5:
Blue- or Red-Skinned Small Potatoes

All potatoes can trace their origins back to the Andes mountains in South America. Today, the International Potato Center in Lima, Peru, recognizes more than 4,500 varieties of potatoes. They're the third most consumed plant on the planet, following wheat and rice, but potatoes have gotten a bad rap for quite some time now. That's partly because we don't eat the most nutritious part of the potato (the skin), and because these tubers have become so processed. The skin of the potato has just as many phytonutrients as broccoli. Many people eat too many of these tubers, but when eaten in moderation, they're a serious brain food. And when the size of the potato is small, like in the case of fingerlings, the ratio of healthy skin skyrockets.

But when those skins are removed and the spuds are cooked in vegetable oils (like soy, corn, and sunflower) loaded with omega-6 fatty acids, you get an entirely different food profile. This abundance of omega-6s elbows out brain-building omega-3 fatty acids and makes us more prone to diabetes.

One particularly rare group of molecules in potatoes, known as kukoamines (otherwise found only in tomatoes and the rare Himalayan goji berry), slow the aging of our brains and lower blood pressure. Potatoes are loaded with vitamin B_6 and folate, both of which eliminate a major marker of depression and heart disease from our blood, homocysteine. B_6 is also a cofactor needed to produce many neurotransmitters, and—last but not least—potato skin is one of the few plant foods that contains iodine, essential for the proper functioning of our thyroid gland. The thyroid is vital for maintaining good moods and one of the first things checked out by psychiatrists when evaluating someone suffering from depression.

The only thing we recommend to avoid, as much as possible, is eating potatoes in the form of french fries or potato chips. Frying potatoes at high heat causes the formation of acrylamide, which is a carcinogen. If you're going to eat potatoes, you should eat them in moderation and whole. Preferably they should be small potatoes with colored skin (more skin per serving and more phytonutrients). Small potatoes have three times as many folates and phytonutrients as mature tubers.

It's true that the top source of the precursor to vitamin A, beta-carotene, in plants is found in the ground—just not in the root, as you might be expecting. Sweet potatoes beat out carrots when it comes to this important nutrient for memory, mood, and immune function.

Rooting for You

Our culture's obsession with processed, fried potatoes means we don't get enough of other roots, which happen to be some of the world's healthiest foods. Plants like turnips, beets, carrots, ginger, radishes, and jicama.

The underground world of roots is colored much like the world of dangling fruits above ground, and this colorful array shows us the breadth of nutrients they contain. (Another clue that some of the most nutritious foods live underfoot is that many of the healthiest leaves are the greens of carrots, beets, and turnips—loaded with essential brain nutrients.)

Carrots—like radishes, beets, and potatoes—come in a rainbow of

TOP 100 REASONS TO AVOID PROCESSED FOODS

One or more rodent hairs are allowed per hundred grams of peanut butter.

colors, and for most of humanity they were purple. The purples in these roots are due to anthocyanins, which have been shown to lower inflammation and quash precancerous cells. These are the same molecules that give blueberries their superfood reputation. These purple root vegetables originated in Afghanistan, but what we commonly think of as a carrot was developed by Dutch breeders in the 1600s. At many farmers' markets today, you can still find the real purple deal. (The Dutch also fed their milking cows carrots to produce bright yellow butter.)

Carrots get their color from carotenoids, and if you eat too many you, too, can turn yellow—a condition known as carotenoderma, where the subcutaneous fat just under your skin contains high concentrations of this nutrient. You can also turn your skin a deep orange with carotenoids like lycopene, the nutrient and pigment found in watermelons, tomatoes, and beets. While harmless, both conditions can take a few weeks to clear up and are most visible in fair-skinned eaters.

How's that for "showing your true colors"?

The Happiness Diet Energy-Boosting Foods

Asparagus	Coffee	Mesclun
Beet greens	Goat cheese	Mustard greens
Broccoli	Green tea	Quinoa
Cabbage	Kale	Red beans
Cauliflower	Lentils	Sweet potatoes
Chocolate	Lettuces	Walnuts

7

Food for Good Mood

When it comes to eating for mood, we want to provide you with foods that don't shock the system but rather help keep you on an even keel throughout the day. We'll want to stay away from highly processed foods, because as you know by now, over time these foods send you down a path that leads to bad health and a lack of mental well-being.

As we've already stated a few times in this book, fat plays an important role in brain health. If you want to eat for mood, it's crucial that you select the fats that are the best for your brain. These are the fats that we find primarily in fish. Also, when we eat whole foods to obtain these nutrients, we get a lot of other vitamins and minerals as a bonus—B-complex vitamins, vitamin D, iodine, and more. All of these nutrients play important roles in keeping you happy throughout the day.

Last but not least, we have to obtain phytochemicals from plants to stay

61 | **TOP 100 REASONS TO AVOID PROCESSED FOODS**

Cooking at home has been linked to longer life spans.

happy. That's because we depend on these nutrients to prevent damage to our brain cells. We also need these nutrients to protect our DNA from damage from our MAD lifestyles. These plant chemicals work in such complex combinations that the science about why they keep people in good moods is just beginning to be thoroughly studied.

What are our favorite picks for great mood foods? We had a tie for numbers one and two.

Top Five Mood Foods
1. Wild salmon and shrimp
2. Cherry tomatoes and watermelon
3. Chile peppers
4. Beets
5. Garlic

Now, let's dive a little deeper into each. . . . First up, let's take a dip in the sea.

Mood Food #1: Wild Salmon and Shrimp

You've no doubt heard enough by this point in the book about the wonders of essential omega-3 fatty acids. But new stories about these special fats come out almost daily, and around the world researchers continue to be stunned by just how important omega-3s are for regulating brain chemistry and optimizing health. When scientists talk about how the Inuit or the Japanese live longer because of their omega-3 consumption, an important fact is left out: These cultures eat fish—not fish oil. Fish is an important

TOP 100 REASONS TO AVOID PROCESSED FOODS

Processed foods speed the process of aging.

source of every Essential Element of Happiness, with the exception of fiber. And two terrifically tasty sources are wild-caught salmon and shrimp.

You know now that fish are such a rich source of omega-3s because the marine food chain begins with phytoplankton. Phytoplankton are tiny plants that drift throughout the world's oceans and lakes. ("Phyto" comes from the Greek word *phyton,* which means plant. "Plankton" comes from the Greek word *planktos,* which means drifter.) They are so small that they cannot be seen with the naked eye, yet they are so numerous that they produce half of our planet's oxygen.

Omega-3s, as you'll soon see, accumulate in nature where high metabolic rates are needed. In fish, that means the need to survive in cold water and travel extreme distances. These are the places in the animal kingdom where—for lack of a better term—miracles happen. And as far as plant life goes, the biggest miracle of all is the act of photosynthesis: the process of converting sunlight into energy, the basis of all life.

In land animals, omega-3s are found most abundantly in the brains of humans. When it comes to incredible feats of endurance, there is no better molecule to rely on than those in the family of shape-shifting, heavy-lifting omega-3s. Prior to migrating thousands of miles, the sandpiper stops at the Bay of Fundy in Canada, where it gorges on shrimp loaded with omega-3s, inducing rapid muscle growth and fueling its flight. The omega-3 DHA is the top fat found in the synaptic connections between our brain cells. These fats are what allow the human heart to contract billions of times over the course of a lifetime without so much as—pun intended—skipping a beat.

63

TOP 100 REASONS TO AVOID PROCESSED FOODS

Got CLA? New research shows this nutrient, found in full-fat, pasture-raised milk, reduces the risk of heart disease by 49 percent. MAD dairy, like skim milk and fat-free yogurt, is stripped of it.

TOP 100 REASONS TO AVOID PROCESSED FOODS

More than eighty thousand chemicals are approved for use in the United States. The vast majority of these have not been studied for their safety—many are found in processed food.

You've likely heard that fish is brain food, but you've likely not heard how wonderful it is for addressing funky moods. When studies compare the mood disorders in different countries, populations that eat the most fish have the lowest rates of depression, bipolar disorder, postpartum depression, and seasonal affective disorder (the winter blues).

Since 1945, the United States' intake of the omega-3 fats found in fish has dropped, while the incidence of depression has increased about twentyfold. This correlation doesn't prove causation, but the mounting evidence that omega-3s are vital for a healthy brain is hard to refute.

Patients diagnosed with depression tend to have lower levels of omega-3s in their blood and 20 to 30 percent less DHA in their brain. A study of one hundred patients in China who had attempted suicide found that they had on average 26 percent lower levels of EPA. People who commit suicide eat less fish, and lower levels of DHA predict the risk of a future suicide attempt.

These fats also seem to play a role in aggression. Young boys with lower levels of omega-3s have more temper tantrums and difficulty falling asleep.

Omega-3s have also been studied as a treatment for a variety of brain-based disorders. A 2008 study found fish oil to have equal efficacy to Prozac in the treatment of depression. Eating omega-3s has also been shown to alleviate the symptoms of depression in more than 60 percent of pregnant women.

Mood Food #2:
Cherry Tomatoes and Watermelon

You might be surprised to learn that the world's most popular berry is actually the tomato. So pull that one out of your pocket the next time your friends are debating whether or not the tomato is a fruit or vegetable.

The tomato originated in the Andes and was transported to Italy by fifteenth-century explorers who encountered the fleshy fruit in Mesoamerica, where the Aztecs called it *tomatl*. Considering its modern-day popularity, it's not surprising that the tomato is also one of the most-studied berries, and today there are more than seven hundred cultivated varieties.

The same compound that makes tomatoes red, lycopene, helps maintain mood by preventing the formation of pro-inflammatory compounds, like interleukin-6, that are associated with depression. This magical molecule is also known to protect against a vast number of cancers (including breast, prostate, and pancreatic). In a study of elderly nuns, those with the most lycopene in their blood lived on average a whopping *eleven years longer* than their sisters with the lowest levels. Organic tomatoes have three times as much of this molecule as conventionally produced ones.

Tomatoes are high in other mood enhancers like folate and magnesium, both used to treat depression. They contain iron, tryptophan, and vitamin B_6: the main ingredients needed by your brain to produce important mood-regulating neurotransmitters like serotonin, dopamine, and norepinephrine. Add to this a high concentration of niacin, vitamin K,

TOP 100 REASONS TO AVOID PROCESSED FOODS

No one studies the long-term "cocktail" affect of artificial ingredients in processed foods. That means many man-made ingredients are surely safe on their own but not when eaten in combination with another synthetic ingredient.

chromium, vitamin C, and potassium, and it makes sense that tomatoes protect us against chronic diseases like diabetes and heart disease. One way these nutrients work is by lowering homocysteine in the blood, a risk factor for depression, heart attacks, and strokes.

Watermelon, too, is red because of lycopene. Did you know that there are more than 1,200 types of watermelon? One is called the Moon and Stars because its black skin is littered with white spots, making it look fantastically like a bright starry night sky out in the countryside. While the rind is bitter, it also contains a lot of citrulline, a nutrient that relaxes blood vessels by activating the same mechanism as the impotency drug Viagra. This compound also helps the brain get rid of the metabolic waste product ammonia, which can damage neurons.

The red flesh of watermelon is bursting with the powerful antioxidant lycopene, much more so actually than the tomato. Lycopene protects our skin from the intense summer sun and kills cancer cells. Studies show you can boost the levels of this important nutrient by up to 40 percent (and beta-carotene by 150 percent) by letting it sit outside the refrigerator at room temperature for several days.

Mood Food #3: Chile Peppers

The chile pepper is a close relative to the tomato berry. The only reason we attach the word *pepper* to the Aztec word *chilli* is because Christopher Columbus believed he'd landed in India and that this spicy fruit was related to Indonesian black peppercorn. It's another of the Americas' great contributions to world cuisine, and all the chile peppers you associate

TOP 100 REASONS TO AVOID PROCESSED FOODS

Frozen pizza often contains phosphate additives—calcium phosphate, disodium phosphate, tricalcium phosphate—that have been linked to lung cancer.

with Indian, Thai, and Chinese foods can be traced back to the mountains of South America.

These fruits are made spicy by the fat-soluble molecule called capsaicin. This molecule is absorbed by fat. If you add chili powder to oil and vinegar, the fat in the oil absorbs all of the capsaicin. It's why a mouthful of guacamole or milk will cool down a burning mouth, while water or beer is unable to put out the fire.

Anthropologists are somewhat confused about why humans enjoy eating food that promotes pain, but sometimes human nature is a few steps ahead of human science. (After all, we've been eating fats on top our salads for eight thousand years, yet only recently did science tell us that this practice helps us absorb the relatively new discovery of science known as vitamins.) While capsaicin sets our mouths on fire, it actually cools our bodies and fights inflammation, blocking the same pathways as aspirin and ibuprofen.

Neuroscientists recently found that the brain is loaded with receptors for capsaicin, which is currently being investigated for its ability to regulate inflammation by influencing the expression of DNA. We also know that our brains respond to the heat of capsaicin by releasing endorphins, natural compounds that are related to morphine and have a calming effect. Capsaicin destroys carcinogens in our food like dimethyl nitrosamine, a preservative in cured meats, and vinyl carbamate, a cancer-causing agent in many pesticides. And capsaicin has been shown to protect the brain during liver failure.

The heat in peppers is measured on the Scoville scale, and the hotter the pepper, the more of this cancer fighter and pain reducer. A habanero clocks in at 350,000 Scoville units, a jalapeño has 8,000, and the lowly old bell pepper has none at all. That's right, the only chile without the health benefits of capsaicin is, coincidentally, the one most commonly encountered with our MADness. It also routinely ends up on the list of the "dirty dozen" of fruits and vegetables compiled by the Environmental Working Group. Capsaicin, like a lot of nutrients in fruit, is a plant's natural defense against pests, and because the bell pepper doesn't contain this spice, the plants are heavily sprayed by growers and are among the most pesticide-contaminated fruits in the grocery store.

Capsaicin plays a role in chile's quite brilliant strategy for spreading its offspring, seeds. Birds' mouths don't have pain receptors that capsaicin binds to, which means that they can eat as many habeneros as their tiny hearts desire and spread the seed far and wide. That's how chiles made their way to the Galapagos Islands long before human settlers arrived.

But the fact that humans are the only mammals that enjoy the burning sensation of capsaicin is another sign of plants' brilliant design, because we've spread these species to all corners of the earth. The receptor for capsaicin in the human brain has led to a second theory about why we like burning our mouths with this compound. When we eat spicy foods, we release the same endorphins as when we exercise. Just like runners report a postworkout high, chile-eaters talk about a soothing, euphoric response to eating extremely spicy food.

Capsaicin is found in the highest concentration in the plant tissue that surrounds the seed, the placenta. By removing this tissue, you can considerably tone down the heat of extreme chiles, like the habanero, while still getting enough of the protective spicy kick. But don't forget that there's

---

TOP 100 REASONS TO AVOID PROCESSED FOODS

Children who eat fast food twice a week are more likely to suffer from asthma.

much, much more to these fruits than capsaicin. Chiles are also great sources of vitamin C (increases absorption of iron), vitamin B_2 (promotes production of your body's natural antioxidants), vitamin B_1 (fights heart disease), vitamin E (protects brain fats), and many others.

Mood Food #4: Beets

A lot of people think of beets as being supersugary, and that's because many eaters were force-fed unpalatable canned versions loaded with as a pagan fruit of ill repute. As a result, growers responded with one of the most successful marketing slogans of all time: An Apple a Day Keeps the Doctor Away.

Eventually Americans had their own native varieties like the McIntosh, the Bottle Greening, the Early Harvest, and the Ladies Favorite of Tennessee. These fruits became popular with early settlers partly because of these varieties' ability to be stored all winter long in root cellars. That is, unless you store them with a bruised fruit, which will release ethylene gas that will speed up decomposition and spoil the whole bushel. That's where we get the term *bad apple*.

Apples are loaded with two important flavonoids: quercetin and epicatechins. These two compounds affect the expression of hundreds of genes influencing mental health, immune function, and the body's ability to process toxins. Epicatechin is transported to the brain, where it blocks monoamine oxidase, an enzyme that recycles neurotransmitters. Catechins, abundantly found in apples, have demonstrated an ability to protect the brain from oxidative damage. Animals pretreated with catechins have less brain damage after being exposed to neurotoxic chemicals or procedures that emulate stroke. These are the same molecules that give green tea its brain-saving reputation. Most of these nutrients are locked away in the skin of the apple, and nowadays that's a problem. All of the popular apple varietals were developed many years ago, and since they're grafted—that is cloned—they've never adapted to predators. That means that one of the most American and most nutritious fruits is also often the most heavily sprayed with pesticides. Always choose organic when picking apples, since the skin is where all the important nutrients are found.

added sugars popularized in the 1950s. It's understandable that people would still have an unfavorable memory of these nutritious root vegetables.

When roasted or boiled, red beets are much less sweet than their canned standbys and impart a deep, earthy flavor. They're delicious pared with goat or blue cheese in a salad and, like good coleslaw, actually taste better after a day in the refrigerator. Beets make a good base for a savory soup that freezes well (see page 189). They can also be shaved with a zester and added raw to salads.

Beets are one of the best sources of the B vitamin folate that is crucial for good mood, memory retrieval, processing speed, and lightning reflexes. Beets are also packed with betaine, which our brain uses to form SAM-e, a natural antidepressant. Uridine, another important nutrient found in these root vegetables, stimulates the production of phosphotidylcholine, a building block of the brain's synaptic connections, helping to increase your mind's processing power. A combination of uridine and omega-3s is as effective as prescription antidepressants in animal studies, and trials of uridine combined with omega-3s are being studied in the treatment of bipolar disorder by Harvard University.

Beets contain another phytonutrient family known as betalains. Two of these compounds, betanin and vulgaxanthin, detoxify the body and reduce inflammation throughout it. Studies on humans have shown that betanins suppress tumor growth through numerous mechanisms, and it's believed that this is mainly done by tamping down enzymes that promote inflammation. As you'll notice, cutting inflammation is something that all the good mood foods have in common.

Mood Food #5: Garlic

Garlic is the star of a family of vegetables known as alliums that include onions, garlic, and leeks. Alliums promote healthy arteries and ensure proper blood flow to the brain. These savory vegetables relax your blood vessels, decreasing your blood pressure, which prevents small strokes in the brain, a major cause of depression and dementia later in life.

Alliums are a top source of a key trace mineral for happiness known as chromium. It's needed for a proper response to the hormone insulin, which

TOP 100 REASONS TO AVOID PROCESSED FOODS

Soy protein, found abundantly in processed foods, has been linked to infertility in women.

helps ensure you're not storing too much sugar as fat. But more than that, it influences the uptake of tryptophan, the precursor to the important neurotransmitter serotonin. It also enhances the release of the neurotransmitter norepinephrine. Chromium supplementation is effective in treating some depressed patients who struggle with low energy and carbohydrate craving. The more sugar in your diet, the more chromium your kidneys excrete, making it harder for insulin to function. Alliums lower blood sugar, and while we don't know exactly why, it may have to do with their high chromium content. Not only that, but the new science shows that allicin in garlic breaks up arterial plaques, essentially reversing heart disease. Garlic also thins blood, further protecting us from heart attack and stroke.

However you slice it, by adding garlic, onions, scallions, or any of the alliums to your daily diet, you'll be protecting your brain, lowering your risk of heart disease, and protecting yourself from the most common forms of cancer (especially of the mouth, throat, colon, and breast).

The Happiness Diet Mood-Boosting Foods

Apples	Lentils	Sprouts
Beets	Garlic	Yogurt
Butter	Lamb	Watermelon
Cherry tomatoes	Milk	Wild salmon
Chile peppers	Onions	Wild shrimp
Cod	Sardines	

8

Shopping and Stocking Your Kitchen

We've just told you what you need to eat to be happy; now it's time to learn how to best choose, where to best buy, and how to select what foods you'll need to get started on your first weeks of living the Happiness Diet. The point of this chapter is to introduce new foods and new ways of doing things into your kitchen. Many of our suggestions will also save you and your family time and money. We've also injected a bunch of practical pointers for preparing these foods. As you're about to see, making fruits and vegetables taste delicious is as simple as tossing some oil and lemon juice on heirloom carrots and cauliflower. Prepare to be dazzled by simplicity of turning produce into delicious, nutritious staples of the Happiness Diet. Don't worry, there's more: Our next chap-

TOP 100 REASONS TO AVOID PROCESSED FOODS

Only 1 percent of obesity is caused by genetics; the rest is caused by diet.

ter will focus on full-out, delicious meal plans for turning the shopping lists we're buying here into a tasty reality.

The Happiness Diet Guide to Perfect Produce

This section is about demystifying the produce section. We are going to show you how to pick produce, easy ways to make it taste splendid, and how to store it—both before and after preparation.

Apples

PICK IT: In the fall through early winter, you can visit greenmarkets to taste heirloom varieties of apples that blow away anything found in most supermarkets.

PREP IT: If you can't find or afford organic yet love apples, soak them first in a solution of white vinegar and water (one part vinegar to three parts water) for an hour or more. Rinse well. This will help get rid of some of the wax and pesticide buildup.

STORE IT: Apples will last for a month in the crisper drawer of your refrigerator. Make sure to keep them in a plastic bag, because they release a natural gas called ethylene that will speed spoilage of other produce.

Artichokes

PICK IT: These spiky vegetables are the flowers of thistle plants. Look for artichokes with scarring, which means the artichokes have been frost kissed and have a concentrated flavor. You can eat the flesh of the leaves, and the interior—the "heart"—lends a tangy, earthy flavor that works in everything from soups to pizzas to eggs.

PREP IT: To prepare a whole artichoke, all you need to do is boil, steam, or braise it and then serve with lemon butter or aioli for dipping.

If you'll be eating the whole artichoke, prep it by cutting about an inch off the top of the bud and trim the spiky tips of the leaves with kitchen scissors. If you don't want to bother with the leaves, trim them off and scrape away the hairy inner layer known as the "choke." Don't trim the stem because it's actually the same delicious material that makes up the heart.

To eat, pull off the leaves one at a time and suck the meaty flesh of the bottom of the leaf. Eventually you'll work your way to the prize, the juicy heart and stem.

STORE IT: Artichoke hearts can be blanched and then packed in plastic bags and frozen for several months.

Asparagus

PICK IT: Usually the first vegetable of spring, asparagus comes in three hues: green, purple, and white. The latter is the most expensive variety and is grown underground so it never develops the green pigment chlorophyll. This practice is done for mostly for appearance and results in a stalk that is less nutrient-dense than green or purple varieties. The best-tasting asparagus has thin, firm stalks and tight tips. If you're on a budget, it's okay not to purchase this vegetable organic. That's because asparagus contains compounds that not only fight disease in humans but repel bugs so that the crops don't need heavy spraying with insecticides.

PREP IT: Asparagus can be steamed, roasted, sautéed, and grilled, and it pairs exceptionally well with lemon, garlic, butter, eggs, and bacon. Be careful not to overcook this vegetable, as the stalks can get mushy quickly.

STORE IT: For storage, wrap the bottom of the stalks in a damp paper towel and place in a plastic bag. It will keep in the crisper drawer for about four days.

Avocado

PICK IT: Most avocados come from California and peak season is summer, though they're available in winter, too. They don't begin to ripen until after they're picked from the tree, so if they are very firm when you buy them, they will benefit from a few days on the kitchen counter wrapped in a paper bag. The best avocados are heavy and firm (but not hard). They're ripe when they just begin to turn soft and feel a tiny bit mushy under the skin to the touch.

PREP IT: This fruit is great in sandwiches and salads and, of course, mashed up as guacamole.

STORE IT: If you have leftover avocado, sprinkle it with lime or lemon juice and store it in a resealable container in the refrigerator to prevent browning. It will last for up to three days.

Beans

PICK IT: There's no better deal at the market than dried beans. At about a dollar per pound (that's six cups cooked), beans are dirt cheap. The most exotic and expensive heirloom varieties—like the Rio Zape available from Rancho Gordo (www.ranchogordo.com)—go for a still-inexpensive five dollars a pound.

PREP IT: Beans are extraordinarily versatile: They can be served whole or pureed, and they marry well with all kinds of flavors. Most types of beans cook more evenly and are more flavorful if soaked ahead of time (ideally overnight). Afterward, they need about an hour atop a stove. Sure, you'll have to plan ahead, but soaking doesn't add much to your actual prep time.

STORE IT: Dried beans look attractive stored in mason jars on the kitchen counter, but they can also go in the freezer—and by keeping your freezer packed to capacity, you'll increase its efficiency. (For more on maximizing the potential of your freezer see "Frozen Assets," page 140.)

TOP 100 REASONS TO AVOID PROCESSED FOODS

The shrimp used for processed food is often laced with carcinogenic chemicals that are banned in the United States.

Beets

PICK IT: Most of us know the deep crimson variety of beet, but this root vegetable can also be white, yellow, orange, or even pink-and-white-striped. Beets can be grated raw and used in salads or slaw; their flavor deepens when boiled, steamed, or roasted. Look for beets that have smooth, unwrinkled skin. The smaller the beet, the sweeter.

PREP IT: When boiling beets, leave the skin on, as it can be rubbed off with minimal effort by running under cool water once tender. Pickled or marinated beets add a tangy sweetness to salads. You can also sauté beet greens like you would Swiss chard or collard greens: use lots of butter and garlic over low heat.

STORE IT: Beets keep for about two weeks in the refrigerator. If you have any leftovers, boil them, cool them, and cut them into slices or cubes—they'll freeze well stored in a plastic bag.

Berries

PICK IT: Blueberries, strawberries, blackberries, and all other berries are only in season for a few fleeting weeks each year. Each of these berries ripen at different times, but generally throughout the spring and summer is when you'll find them. Buy organic when you can. Luckily, they freeze well, allowing you to enjoy their summery flavors all year long. When buying fresh berries, tilt the container—the fruit should roll around, not stick together. You can buy frozen berries in the winter months, which have about the same nutrient value as fresh and tend to be less expensive.

STORE IT: Keep fresh berries in the container they came in (it promotes air circulation) and use them within a few days. To freeze them, arrange individually on a cookie sheet unwashed (additional moisture will alter their texture in the freezer—just remember to wash them before use). After freezing, remove berries from the cookie sheet and store in bags.

Broccoli

PICK IT: Usually sold as one large, compact head, broccoli also comes in a more exotic variety called "sprouting broccoli" that consists of several smaller heads and sometimes comes in exotic hues like purple. No matter what type you choose, the florets should be firm and evenly colored, with no yellowing, and with stalks that are not slimy, withered, or discolored.

PREP IT: Most people steam or sauté broccoli, but it's delicious tossed with olive oil, garlic, salt, and freshly ground black pepper and roasted in the oven until the edges begin to caramelize. Or try substituting steamed broccoli (let it cool first) for basil in pesto.

STORE IT: Broccoli should be stored in an open plastic bag; it will stay fresh in your refrigerator's crisper for up to five days.

Brussels Sprouts

PICK IT: These crucifers look like small heads of cabbage and are usually sold loose, but they actually grow on a thick stalk in clusters of twenty to forty. The smaller the sprout, generally, the more mild and tender it is.

PREP IT: To prepare, simply sauté in butter with salt and fresh cracked pepper. Taste frequently to ensure that you don't overcook, as these vegetables soften easily and are best with a bit of crunch.

STORE IT: They taste best if eaten within a few days of purchase; they start to get mushy after five days in the refrigerator.

Carrots

PICK IT: Baby carrots might be convenient, but they're not as tasty or nutritious as the whole variety. The miniature versions are actually big carrots that were blemished that growers whittle down and bag as "babies." Processing, however, causes them to lose flavor and nutrients. Instead, buy carrots whole when they're in season, typically October

TOP 100 REASONS TO AVOID PROCESSED FOODS

Fumes of diacetyl, a chemical that for years gave microwave popcorn its buttery flavor, cause severe lung disease.

through April, and look for them in a variety of colors like white, yellow, pink, red, and purple. Carrot greens are one of the most nutritious greens around and can be detached and eaten on their own.

PREP IT: Carrots are sugary and add sweetness to soups, stews, and stir-fries. They're delicious eaten raw, especially when sliced and topped with a drizzle of olive oil, lemon juice, salt, and freshly ground black pepper—a great fresh side for any meal. Carrots are also delicious glazed. To do so, slice and simmer a pound (about seven) in a cup of water with a few tablespoons of butter until the carrots are tender and the liquid has reduced. Salt and pepper to taste and experiment by adding fresh herbs, sautéed onions, or lemon zest. Roasting and tossing carrots into a vinaigrette is another option.

STORE IT: If you're storing carrots for more than a few days (they keep for a few weeks), remove the tops because they speed deterioration.

Cauliflower

PICK IT: This head of florets is found freshest in the fall and winter and can be eaten raw or cooked. Raw cauliflower is best when it tastes sweet, but this flavor profile disappears long before you can visibly see cauliflower starting to go bad. To check for sweetness, smell the head. If you detect a sour odor, look for another bunch (the sour odor goes away when cooked). Avoid precut florets, because they'll be dried out and their taste compromised. Today, many grocers are starting to sell miniature cauliflower that comes in yellow, white, and purple, and each has a slightly different flavor. We recommend experimenting as often as possible.

PREP IT: Soak all cauliflower upside down in salted water for a few minutes to draw out bugs. An easy and delicious way to prepare cauliflower is to roast it for thirty to forty minutes at 350 degrees with some butter, and then toss it in a light vinaigrette (see page 218).

STORE IT: Store it whole for up to a week in your refrigerator's crisper.

Chile Peppers

PICK IT: From mild (poblano) to five-alarm hot (habanero), chile peppers are at their peak from late summer to early fall. All chiles start out green and turn red when mature. So ancho chiles, for example, are simply fully matured (and dried) poblano peppers.

PREP IT: If you have a lot you haven't used, you can dry them on a cookie sheet in a warm oven on the lowest setting of 100 to 150 degrees for six hours, or on a windowsill for one to two days.

STORE IT: Store fresh peppers in a plastic bag in your refrigerator's crisper drawer for up to a week. Dried chiles have a more concentrated flavor and, if kept dry, will last indefinitely. If a recipe calls for fresh chiles, you'll need to first reconstitute your dried ones by soaking them in warm water. Peppers also freeze well and will last up to a year or more in your freezer.

Corn

PICK IT: There are hundreds of varieties of corn, but Americans generally tend to cook with sweet corn, which is in season roughly from May

---

TOP 100 REASONS TO AVOID PROCESSED FOODS

Big Tobacco owns many of America's most popular processed-food brands, like Nabisco and Kraft.

through September. The freshest corn will have plump, bright kernels that you can pop with a fingernail.

PREP IT: Corn can be boiled in salted water for about four minutes. Or soak corn in the husk and throw it on the grill for about five to ten minutes. Roll the husk back and use it as a handle. Keep the used cobs to make a stock for soups or chowders.

STORE IT: As soon as corn is picked, its sugars turn to starches (which may be why many people describe the pleasure of eating freshly cooked corn on the cob as a near-religious experience). So sweet corn should be used as soon as possible, though it does last a week or more in the refrigerator. A better option, though, if you know you're not going to eat it immediately, is to blanch the corn and remove and then freeze the kernels (they'll keep for up to a year).

Cucumbers

PICK IT: Buy organic, unwaxed cucumbers in season from May through July.

PREP IT: Cucumbers benefit from being salted to soften their texture and to prevent them from watering down dishes. To do so, halve a cucumber, scoop out the seeds, and sprinkle the flesh of each half with sea salt (about half a teaspoon). Place the halves in a colander and let sit for thirty minutes. Afterward, rinse off the salt and gently squeeze the halves to remove excess water. Pat dry, slice, and use for salad.

STORE IT: These store well for weeks uncovered in your crisper.

TOP 100 REASONS TO AVOID PROCESSED FOODS

Like tobacco companies before them, processed-food manufacturers now offer "healthier" versions of products that are no better at preventing disease than the foods that preceded them. In other words, low-tar cigarettes equal low-fat cookies.

Fresh Herbs

PICK IT: Fresh herbs not only brighten the flavor of food but also boost nutrient content. Many of the varieties you'll reach for most often, like basil, tarragon, mint, oregano, thyme, parsley, cilantro, dill, and rosemary, can be grown in containers on your windowsill, allowing you to pinch off just what you need for a recipe, and then watch it grow right back.

PREP IT: If you want to use fresh herbs in a recipe that calls for dried, the general rule is to use three times as much. Fresh herbs are also amazing in salads.

STORE IT: Herbs you buy at a market should be wrapped in a slightly damp paper towel (to help keep them from drying out) and placed in a perforated plastic bag in the refrigerator's crisper where they'll store for up to a week.

Durable herbs like rosemary and thyme—the ones that can stand up to cooking—can be placed in plastic storage bags and frozen for up to a year. More tender herbs like basil and cilantro, which are added at the end of cooking because they wilt and brown quickly, generally won't freeze as well but are still usable for soups and stews.

Another option is to mince the herbs and pour into ice trays with water and freeze. These cubes can be dropped into sauces and soups as needed. Or you can freeze spices like basil as pesto. It, too, can be frozen in cubes and used as you need it for sandwiches, pasta, or whatever you see fit.

Garlic

PICK IT: Raw garlic is pungent, and cooking it brings out the bulb's sweetness. Buy garlic that is firm to the touch. If it's shriveled or spongy, the bulb is about to sprout and will be bitter. Crush or mince garlic cloves to boost the content of allicin, a compound that strengthens immunity.

PREP IT: Sautéing garlic in butter or olive oil is a great way to start most any dish that you cook in a skillet—from scrambled eggs to stir-fries.

STORE IT: Store garlic in a cool, dry, dark place to prevent sprouting. Summer garlic lasts a few weeks, while dry winter garlic will last months.

Green Beans

PICK IT: One of the few varieties of legumes we eat fresh, green beans (also known as string beans) come in a range of colors like yellow and purple. Ripe green beans will be brightly colored and will snap cleanly when bent.

PREP IT: Boil or blanch beans carefully, as they overcook easily and can become mushy. A good trick is throwing them in a bowl of ice water as soon as you are finished blanching them to stop them from cooking and to preserve a nice bright color—a trick that works with well with broccoli and asparagus, too. Beans pickle nicely (do them just as you would cucumbers, or they can be pickled together). Aside from snacks, pickles are great additions to salads and sandwiches.

STORE IT: Uncooked, unused beans last about a week or so in the crisper of your refrigerator.

Greens

PICK IT: Each green—from arugula to Swiss chard—has its own set of happiness-promoting, disease-fighting phytochemicals, which is why you should eat a wide variety of them. Opt for organic whenever you can. In general, the smaller the leaves, the more tender and mild they'll be.

PREP IT: Many of the nutrients found in leaves are fat-soluble, so you should always eat greens with fats—whether it's cheese, olive oil, or butter. The only trick to eating greens is dressing them properly (store-bought salad dressings are full of preservatives and wildly overpriced). Tougher leaves like kale can be softened by first blanching or sautéing in butter and then dressing just like you would a salad.

STORE IT: Wrap greens in a paper towel before storing in a plastic bag in the crisper. This will absorb moisture that accelerates spoilage.

Lemon and Lime

PICK IT: Look for fruit with thinner skin because that means more pulp and hence more juice. If you can find organic, it's worth the premium, because the zest of the skin is rich with limonoids that fight all kinds of disease.

PREP IT: Acidic and bright, lemons and limes are arguably as versatile as the allium family. They can be used in marinades as a tenderizer; to perk up fish, add a kick to drinks, or cut the spice out of dishes; as the base of a salad dressing; or as a stand-in for vinegar.

STORE IT: Citrus juice freezes well whole and lasts for a year or more. You can also pour it into ice cube trays; when frozen, store the loose cubes in plastic freezer bags.

Mushrooms

PICK IT: There are thousands of varieties of mushrooms, and most specialty grocers offer a good selection. Cremini mushrooms are similar in

TOP 100 REASONS TO AVOID PROCESSED FOODS

In August 2011, Cargill recalled 36 million pounds of ground turkey products because of concern that they were contaminated with *Salmonella* Heidelberg—a multidrug-resistant strain.

size to the standard white button mushrooms but are firmer and more flavorful, making them a good all-purpose choice for salads and soups. Portobellos are larger relatives of the cremini and are great grilled. Shiitake mushrooms have a spongy texture and woodsy flavor that lends well to stir-fries or being tossed with earthy grains like barley. Enoki mushrooms are long, thin, and mild and are common in Asian cuisines (they're often added to miso soup). Lastly, maitake mushrooms (also known as hen of the woods) have large ruffled caps and a savory flavor—they're delicious pan-fried until crispy.

PREP IT: The flavor of mushrooms will be strongest if you cook them slowly in a manner that draws out some of their moisture (like oven roasting). Mushrooms contain a special fiber called chitin, which prevents them from turning mushy when cooked—making them perfect for use in soups and stews.

STORE IT: Mushrooms should be used as soon as possible but will keep in the refrigerator for up to about five days. Place them in a paper bag or wrap them in a paper towel to absorb excess moisture and prevent spoilage.

Onions and Shallots

PICK IT: These alliums grow underground like root vegetables, but they're much more versatile and are staples of nearly all of the world's most influential cuisines. There are two types of large globe onions: "storage" and "sweet." Storage onions like Spanish and yellow onions are allowed to dry for several months before taking them to market, which gives them a

TOP 100 REASONS TO AVOID PROCESSED FOODS

The reason 7UP with antioxidants is sold is because its manufacturer wants us to believe this sugary soda is healthier than any other sugary soda.

concentrated, spicy flavor. Sweet onions like Walla Walla, Maui, and Vidalia appear in markets in summer and, because of their higher water content, don't keep as long. Shallots are a milder, more tender relative of the storage onion and are available year-round.

The sulfur compounds that protect onions and shallots from pests also cause them to require less pesticides in conventional farming—so buying organic isn't essential if you're on a budget.

PREP IT: Members of the allium family contain disease-fighting sulfur compounds that are released when cut into and bring tears to many of our eyes. The sharper your knife, the fewer sulfur compounds will be released because less surface area of the onion is disturbed. You can protect your eyes by chilling onions and shallots before dicing, which makes the eye-watering compounds less volatile.

STORE IT: Both varieties should be stored outside the refrigerator in a cool, dark place where they'll last for weeks. The only types of onion that should be stored in the fridge are scallions and spring onions that are harvested fresh. Keep them in a plastic bag in the crisper and they'll last about four or five days.

Oranges

PICK IT: Most of the oranges you see at grocery stores are navel oranges from Florida or California, which are meant for eating, not juicing (they produce only a small amount of juice, and it turns bitter quickly). Other common varieties include Valencia, Clementine, and blood oranges; most are available year-round but reach their peak from December through May. It's best to buy organic, as conventional oranges are often injected with artificial dye to give them a uniform color.

PREP IT: Orange zest, though less versatile than lemon or lime zest, can be used in stir-fries, marinades, and desserts.

STORE IT: Oranges can be stored in the refrigerator for up to two weeks.

Pears

PICK IT: Pears should be slightly firm at purchase, and their necks should yield to gentle pressure from your finger.

PREP IT: The options for sugary, ripe pears are almost endless. They're great in salads with pungent, salty cheeses like Gorgonzola. Or in pies, baked with molasses or brown sugar. They're also great grilled or poached.

STORE IT: Store pears at room temperature until they've fully ripened (placing them in a paper bag speeds the process). Once ripe, they can last in the crisper for about five days (make sure they're stored in a perforated bag because they need air circulation or they'll go brown). Like apples, pears release ethylene gas that speeds the spoilage of other produce, so keep them separated. Store them away from strong-smelling foods, too, because pears absorb odors easily.

To freeze pears, core and slice them. Then simmer the slices for a few minutes in simple syrup. (To make simple syrup, combine one part sugar with one part water and boil; let cool before using.) Let the pear-syrup solution cool, add a bit of lemon juice, and then pour into plastic bags and freeze. They'll keep for more than a year.

Potatoes

PICK IT: There are thousands of varieties of potatoes. Any potato you buy should be firm and smooth, with no sprouts. Avoid spuds with green on the skin—this could indicate the presence of solanine, a neurotoxin produced by exposure to light. Most nutrients are found in and just below the skin, and that's why you should consider buying organic—potatoes are among the top twelve foods most likely to contain pesticide residue (which accumulates in their skins).

PREP IT: Boiling potatoes, like the Red Bliss, have waxy skins that hold up well to boiling water—but they can become sticky and gooey when mashed. Baking potatoes, like the russet, have dry, coarse skin and mealy flesh that becomes light and fluffy when baked, mashed, or fried. Some varieties, like Yukon Gold and Peruvian Blue, have properties of both baking and boiling potatoes and can be used for either purpose.

STORE IT: Store potatoes in burlap or a paper bag (not plastic; potatoes need to breathe) in a cool, dark place and use them within about a month. Don't store them in the refrigerator, because the cool temperature will cause the tuber to convert its starch to sugar, altering the flavor.

Summer Squash/Zucchini

PICK IT: Zucchini, the best-known variety of summer squash, is 95 percent water. As such, it will be most flavorful when you cook out that moisture. Choose smaller squashes: They'll have less water and more flavor. You should consume zucchini with the skin on, so be sure to buy organic when possible.

PREP IT: Squash blossoms, the edible yellow-orange flowers, are too delicate and perishable to be found at the store but may show up at the greenmarket—they're delicious stuffed with ricotta, battered, and flash-fried. Like cucumber, squash can be salted to draw out some moisture before eating raw. Zucchini can stand in for cucumbers when making pickles or be pureed to use in baked goods like breads and cakes. (A simple, amazing recipe is tossing a few yellow and green squash into a mandoline on the smallest setting and then tossing the resulting "spaghetti" slices with olive oil, lemon juice, and salt and pepper.)

STORE IT: Squash will last a few weeks in your crisper.

Tomatoes

PICK IT: Buy organic tomatoes when possible, as research shows they have three times more of the cancer-fighting compound lycopene than conventional varieties. Check your farmers' market for plum tomatoes (great for making sauce), cherry tomatoes (sweeter and perfect for snacking), and heirloom tomatoes (great for salads, sandwiches, and just about anything else) in all sorts of colors, like the deep pink Brandywine and the striped Green Zebra. Always buy in season.

PREP IT: Slice tomatoes with a serrated knife to prevent bruising and a messy presentation.

STORE IT: Don't store at temperatures below fifty-five because they'll lose flavor. Tomato puree and sauce—but not whole fruit—hold up very well in the freezer.

Turnips

PICK IT: This bulbous root is sweet and mild, and its leafy greens are edible. Small turnips are generally sweeter and less fibrous.

PREP IT: Turnips can be cooked in a covered saucepan with just a little butter and salt and then served whole, mashed, or pureed. Turnips can also be steamed or roasted whole with their greens still attached; serve them with butter and salt.

STORE IT: Store turnips with greens detached in a plastic bag in the refrigerator for up to two weeks; they get bitter with age . . . like some people.

Watermelon

PICK IT: When shopping for a watermelon, look for one with a creamy white or yellowish spot. That's where the watermelon rested on the ground, and it's an indication that the melon was allowed to ripen before harvest.

PREP IT: While watermelon is usually enjoyed on its own, it has many other uses. It can be cubed and juiced. You can either drink it straight or use it as a mix for cocktails or as a base for gazpacho. (Some swear by freezing the juice in ice cube trays and using the cubes in iced tea.) The rind—which contains citrulline, an amino acid that helps relax blood vessels—is also edible. Because it can be bitter, most people eat it pickled in vinegar, sugar, and spices. (If you plan on eating the rind, buy an organic watermelon, since rinds are where pesticide residues accumulate.)

STORE IT: Store at room temperature for most nutrient bang for the buck, which means up to a week or more. Cover and refrigerate leftovers for up to a week or turn into juice.

· · · · · · · · · ·

Now that you're a master of picking, prepping, and storing produce, let's move on to some other happy foods—meats—and how to buy them economically and smartly.

How to Buy a Whole Animal

If you want to save money on pasture-raised, grass-fed meats, cut out the middleman—your grocer. Buying direct from the farmer is simple. All you need to do is wrangle some like-minded friends (colleagues, school parents, or neighbors) and decide how much meat your collective group can reasonably freeze (meat keeps well for about six months).

At Local Harvest (www.localharvest.org), you can search for local grass farmers, as they like to call themselves, by entering your zip code. Many sell whole and half animals at steep discounts from the farmers' market or gourmet grocer. You'll be exposed to a bevy of flavorful cuts that you won't often find at the regular meat counter, such as short ribs and pork shoulder.

Buying a whole pastured pig will net about 160 pounds of meat and will set you back about three to five dollars per pound. A grass-fed steer produces about 560 pounds of meat at anywhere from two to six dollars a pound. Lamb is a bit more expensive at six to nine dollars per pound (a whole animal will provide about thirty-five pounds of meat). The meat will come separated and packed ready for storage in the freezer. Many of these farmers also sell pasture-raised chickens, ducks, geese, and turkey, all of which are often heritage varieties that are much more flavorful than their mass-produced counterparts. You can even use the bones to create stock for soup or sauces.

How to Join a CSA

Community-supported agriculture (or CSA) is a term that describes how a community and a local farm can form a mutually beneficial relationship. Members pay an annual share that supports the farm, and in return they receive weekly allocations of fresh produce. Unlike shopping at a grocery store or greenmarket, you don't get much say in the produce you receive each week, which is what a lot of people actually enjoy about the practice—you learn how to cook in the way that used to be second nature to cooks just a few generations ago: seasonally. If you get a surplus of, say, butternut squash, you'll have to come up with creative ways to cook it all or preserve it for later (like making squash puree and then freezing it).

CSA prices vary but generally cost between $450 to $600 per year for a full share of produce (enough for two to four people); half shares with a more limited selection are often available for smaller households. It might sound like a lot of money at first, but most people find that in reality it's often cheaper than buying produce at the grocery store.

Frozen Assets

No other luxury of modernity can help you save money on groceries more than your freezer. It allows you to buy food in bulk and use it as the need arises. When frozen correctly, fresh fish and meat can last from six months to more than a year.

This appliance is also essential in cutting down the estimated six hundred dollars of fresh food the average American family tosses out each year in the garbage. When you have leftovers or fresh produce that's about to spoil, a freezer can extend those foods indefinitely. It's also a great way to store cheap, seasonal produce for off-season months. Apples and pears, for example, are bargains during the fall, and to freeze them all you have to do is blanch them, then store them in plastic bags in simple syrup, and they'll last for more than a year.

Butter, cheese, lemon juice, stock, and pesto all freeze well. Chill them in ice cube trays, store the cubes in labeled plastic bags, and use as needed in sauces and soups. To prevent freezer burn, make sure the containers have as little air inside as possible; for beans or grains, cover with a layer of water or oil to prevent the same. Bread stores well as a whole loaf and can be reheated on low in the oven. Store leftovers in single-serving containers so that they can be used as needed.

Frozen foods tend to look alike so, again, be sure to label everything and be specific ("beef and bean chili" is more useful than simply "chili") and include the date. You want your freezer to run as efficiently as possible, and it does this when it's full because that translates into less air exchange when it's opened and closed. Frozen gallons of water and dry beans are cheap and effective ways of filling up freezer space.

The most energy-efficient freezers are chest freezers that can be found for as little as a few hundred dollars at your appliance store. They've become so efficient, in fact, that they'll set you back only about $20 in

TOP 100 REASONS TO AVOID PROCESSED FOODS

Residues of more than seventy pesticides have been found in individual boxes of cereal.

annual energy costs. If you don't have garage space to store one, consider locating it somewhere in your kitchen and using its top surface as extra counter space. You can attach a cutting board to its lid and use it as a prep station.

Buying Grass-Fed Butter

Think of butter as the whole grain of cooking fats. It has a long list of nutrients—including vitamin A, vitamin D, folate, magnesium, and vitamin B_{12}—not found in vegetable oils (and, yes, that includes olive oil). Grass-fed butter is even healthier. It has more of those aforementioned nutrients, plus loads of omega-3 fatty acids and CLA.

In short, the more fresh grass a cow eats, the more nutritious its milk and butter. That's why aficionados swear by butter that comes from spring- and early-summer–fed milking cows. It's bright and yellow because the cream is loaded with beta-carotene, the precursor to vitamin A. Because butter keeps for up to a year or more in your freezer, you can stock up in the spring for a year's supply.

Find a local grass-fed dairy farm at www.eatwild.com or at your local farmers' market. Many mainstream grocery stores as well are starting to carry products like Organic Valley's Pasture Butter, which is produced regionally by collectives of small, independently owned organic family farms.

Online Resources for Buying Locally

Locally grown produce is often picked the same morning it is purchased—which means the most brain- and heart-protecting nutrients possible still reside inside it. Shopping locally also supports the small farms in your neighborhood. Buying at a neighborhood greenmarket is an easy way to start buying local foods, if you have one available nearby:

There are more than five thousand of them operating in the United States, an 84 percent jump from just a decade ago.

But if you don't have one in your community, you may still be able to buy fresh, healthy food directly from a farm. The same group we mentioned earlier that could help you find a local CSA, Local Harvest, maintains a national database of farms and farmers' markets, all searchable by zip code at localharvest.org.

If you're curious about how your community compares to others in terms of its numbers of farms and markets, the USDA has an interactive map at maps.ers.usda.gov/FoodAtlas.

PUTTING UP PICKLES

Pickling is an easy way to preserve in-season produce like cucumbers, beets, green beans, and chile peppers to eat out of season for pennies on the dollar. It's an art perfected by mothers and grandmothers that almost disappeared in the age of convenience, but it's making a comeback as more and more people reconnect with fresh food. Pickles are great, of course, as snacks, but they can also be chopped up and added to salads, sauces, and condiments.

All you need to get started are a few basic fresh ingredients, a pot of boiling water, and glass canning jars. We suggest beginning with fresh dill, garlic, jalapeños (for a not-too-over-the-top spicy kick), kosher salt, and vinegar. You'll also need a glass canning jar like those sold by Ball.

Disinfect a jar by gently dropping it (and its lid) in boiling water. Next, boil a 50/50 mixture of white vinegar and water with a cup of salt per liter for the pickling brine. While that's on the stove, stuff the jar with the vegetables you want to pickle, leaving ¼ inch of room at the top. Pack the veggies as tightly as possible. Once the salt has dissolved in the brine, remove the liquid from the heat and then pour over your pickles. Store the jars in a cool dry place. Once you have the basics down, you can experiment with many different flavor combinations. Try adding mustard seeds, coriander, or peppercorns. Pickle sweeter produce like watermelon rind (amazing in salads) or grapes with sugar, salt, cinnamon, and black peppercorn. Pickles take about eight weeks to develop and last indefinitely.

Label Decoder

We want you off all processed foods, ideally. Yet people still find premade packaged foods convenient, and we get that. But never buy anything processed without a careful glance at the ingredients. The difference between two brands can mean the presence or absence of toxic preservatives or natural food colorants as opposed to artificial ones. Labels can be really confusing, and that's why we've compiled lists here of terms you should watch out for, as well as seek out.

Terms to Be Wary Of

NATURAL: For the most part, this label is completely meaningless and unregulated. The only time it's enforced is in the case of meat and poultry, and then it's regulated by the USDA. Still, "natural" applies only to the finished product. It means that meat or poultry after slaughter must contain "no artificial ingredient or added color" and be "only minimally processed" (a process that does not fundamentally alter the raw product), but there's no restriction on what chemicals and hormones animals receive while the animals are alive.

NO ARTIFICIAL INGREDIENTS/MADE WITH NATURAL FLAVORINGS: This claim is even less regulated than "natural." A product could boast this on the package and still be full of highly processed additives that technically originated from a natural ingredient (such as soybeans or corn).

LIGHTLY SWEETENED: You might see this claim on the label of a seemingly healthy beverage like Newman's Own lemonade. Unfortunately, that drink could still contain as much as eighteen grams of sugar (like the aforementioned brand)—that's four tablespoons of sugar in one glass.

ORGANIC: Why is this on our "wary" list? Most times, this is a worthwhile label to seek out. It means the product you're purchasing is free of synthetic pesticides, hormones, and other nasty chemicals that as a group have been linked to brain disorders, weight gain, and a laundry list of other problems. For meat to be labeled organic, it means that at least 30 percent of the animal's diet was on pasture.

But when it comes to farmed fish—namely farmed salmon—this term is meaningless. The farmers may use chemicals to manage parasites and feed their fish nonorganic food, and those pollutants can ultimately end up in the water. Studies have shown that farmed organic salmon is loaded with PCBs and dioxins.

MADE WITH ORGANIC INGREDIENTS: Some organic ingredients are better than none, but this claim misses the whole point of eating organic—which is to avoid foods grown using pesticides. A product can use the "made with organic ingredients" label if at least 70 percent of its ingredients are organic. Foods with the green-and-white USDA seal meet the more stringent requirement that they be at least 95 percent organic.

MADE WITH REAL FRUIT: You might see this claim on a toaster pastry, fruit snack, or juice container when in reality the only "real fruit" the product contains is a negligible amount of processed pear concentrate.

MADE WITH WHOLE WHEAT: This term can mean that a small fraction of the product actually contains whole wheat. If you're looking for whole wheat bread, check the ingredients. Items are listed in descending order of content, most to least. "Whole wheat flour" should be the first ingredient and the package should say "100 percent whole wheat."

HIGH IN FIBER: Some processed foods advertise this claim when in fact they're pumped with fillers like bamboo or chitosan (made from the skeletons of insects and shellfish). These ingredients boost fiber content and often improve shelf life, but they're not the type of fiber that coevolved with your stomach to keep you thin and prevent disease.

TOP 100 REASONS TO AVOID PROCESSED FOODS

Today, more kids recognize McDonald's Golden Arches than the Christian cross.

TRANS FAT FREE: This claim means that the product contains half a gram of trans fats or less per serving. This means that a standard box of Ritz Crackers contains up to fourteen grams of trans fats.

HORMONE FREE: The USDA already prohibits the use of hormones in pork and poultry products, so if you see this label on, say, deli ham, the manufacturer is stating the obvious in an attempt to sound "natural." Hormone-free claims are important when it comes to dairy products, however.

A GOOD SOURCE OF: This phrase technically means a product contains more than 10 percent but less than 20 percent of the recommended daily allowance of a particular nutrient per serving. It's misleading, because this label is applied to sugared foods like breakfast cereals—tricking consumers into thinking what they're buying is healthy when in fact it isn't.

Terms to Seek Out

U.S. GRASS-FED: In response to consumer demand, the USDA introduced a "Grass Fed" label in 2009. It requires that an animal eat grass throughout its entire life, but mandates access to the outdoors only during the grass-growing season. This means that, in the winter months, an animal may be confined to a barn and fed forage. The American Grassfed Association has more rigorous standards. In order for a product to acquire its seal, "animals . . . be maintained at all times on range, pasture, or in paddocks with at least 75% forage cover or unbroken ground for their entire lives" and that farmers "must support humane animal welfare, handling, transport and slaughter."

NATURALLY RAISED: The USDA allows this label on meat products that "have been raised entirely without growth promotants, antibiotics, and have never been fed animal by-products." But there are no requirements about access to the outdoors and pasture.

HUMANELY RAISED: This label ensures that animals are treated gently to minimize stress, are allowed to engage in natural behaviors (pigs can root; chickens can dust bathe), and are not given feed with growth hormones or antibiotics. Your best bet is to look for an actual seal (not just a claim on the front of the package) provided by a third-party certifier like Humane Farm Animal Care.

FED AN ALL-VEGETARIAN DIET: The meat industry generates millions of tons of animal by-products every year, and most of it—including trimmings and condemned carcasses—gets recycled into animal feed for chickens and pigs. If you see on a package of bacon or eggs that the animal was fed a vegetarian diet, you can take comfort in the fact that "condemned carcasses" weren't on the menu. Just be aware that this label doesn't specify exactly what's in the nonmeat feed: It could include waste products, like plastic.

FREE RANGE/CAGE FREE: The terms "cage free" and "free range" ensure your grocery store dollars don't support hens being raised packed in cages. Unfortunately, the term "cage free" doesn't mean hens have access to outdoors, although they usually have room to walk around and perch. "Free range" hens technically have access to the outdoors with fresh air and sunlight, but there's no rule yet that ensures that this is a grassy field and not a concrete lot. The only way to truly know for sure how your chicken or egg was raised is to get to know your farmer, which is why farm stands and farmers' markets are so important.

NO rBGH: This claim, found on dairy products, means the milk was produced without the use of the hormone rBGH (also known as rBST). Milk from cows given this adulterant have higher levels of a hormone that is linked to cancer in humans.

GMO-FREE: Genetically modified organisms (GMOs) are developed through gene-splicing—a process that can implant fish genes into blueberries. The goal is to create high-yield, pest-resistant crops that grow quickly. Opponents of GMOs argue that the crops threaten biodiversity, haven't been proven safe for human consumption, and

TOP 100 REASONS TO AVOID PROCESSED FOODS

The cost of the corn in an average box of cornflakes accounts for one-tenth of the final retail price. Nine-tenths is markup.

could cross-contaminate organic crops. Europe banned the vast majority of GMOs, but in the United States, about 90 percent of soy plants and 75 percent of corn are genetically modified. GMO-free products have been grown by farmers who do not use this controversial practice.

ORGANIC: When you buy organic, you're choosing foods made without chemical fertilizers, pesticides, growth hormones and antibiotics, and GMOs. They also weren't irradiated—a common practice where produce, meats, and other raw ingredients are zapped to kill pests and slow spoilage. A product can use the word *organic* on its label and/or display the USDA's green-and-white organic seal if at least 95 percent of its ingredients are organic. Many small farms practice organic farming methods but don't bother with the expense of getting officially certified. The best way to know for sure is to ask.

MARINE STEWARDSHIP COUNCIL (MSC)-CERTIFIED: Fish products that carry this seal (a blue fish with a checkmark) have demonstrated that they follow sustainable practices designed to minimize the environmental impact of fishing and keep fish stocks healthy.

WILD ALASKAN: Any salmon labeled Alaskan is wild because the state does not allow fish farming, which explains why they still have healthy wild stocks.

FAIR TRADE: Fair trade means that the workers that produce the crops used to make your food are paid a living wage and that they learn and practice environmentally sustainable methods of farming.

Now that we know where our food is coming from and we know what to buy, let's look at what a couple of weeks of eating happy will look like.

Happy Meal Plans—Two Weeks of Simple, Tasty, Feel-Good Menus

Here it is. It's what we've been building up to how and what to eat, spelled out and made simple. Two weeks. Every meal. Every snack.

The menu plan below is built on the Happiness Diet principles:

- **Eliminate processed foods.** They make us fat and unhappy. Do this and immediately you can stop worrying about eating too much sugar and refined carbs, trans fats, artificial food colorings, and toxins lurking in your food packaging.

- **Balance your fats.** Every day that follows gives you a mix of omega-3s, CLA, monounsaturated, and saturated fats. Excess omega-6s are minimized as long as you get your meat from grass-fed sources. Use traditional fats like butter, lard, and olive oil. By using these fats, you'll ensure that you'll always be getting all the happy-brain-making, fat-soluble nutrients like vitamins A, D, E, and K you need.

- **Eat fish at least twice a week.** Incorporate a variety of seafood so you maximize your intake of brain-essential nutrients like iodine, zinc, B_{12}, and copper, all while increasing your intake of long-chain omega-3s, DHA, and EPA.

- **Pile on the produce.** Eat a variety of colorful fruits and vegetables as the foundation of your diet. Plants are our form of portion control. In every day of the menu plan, we incorporate leafy greens and a bounty of vegetables so you constantly are replenishing folates, vitamin C, and other important phytonutrients.

- **Focus on nutrients, not calories.** Quality, not quantity, is what counts when it comes to feeding your brain right.

- **Ditch the soda and fruit juice.** Drink water, coffee, tea, wine, and beer. Don't overdo any of the above; the old adage "Everything in moderation" continues to be wise advice.

A few key pointers for what follows. We count on you to follow a few rules. They are:

Rule #1. Eat more plants than meat or dairy.

Rule #2. MAD portions get reversed; instead of a giant portion of refined carbs (for example, pasta, pizza, or bread) eat unrefined (read: whole) vegetables.

Rule #3. Try to eat slower, chew a little longer, and savor the flavors of your food a lot more. If you are used to processed foods, your palate is accustomed to those flavors. Recalibration takes a little time.

Rule #4. Nearly everyone has a sweet tooth, and most of us enjoy dessert. We just encourage you not to make it an everyday thing. They call carbs and sugar comfort foods for a reason, so pick one day a week and enjoy small portions of these treats.

That's it for the rules.

Some of you are experienced cooks, so use what follows as a launching point for your own "takes" on these dishes. Others of you might have minimal knowledge of cooking. That's okay. Nothing below is fancy; it requires no more than a few minutes of prep time and no special tools. The recipes employ what we think is the only food processor you'll ever need—YOU.

Not sure you want to do this for two weeks? Maybe you want to start smaller, but are not sure where and how to begin? Just decide based on where you are starting from.

If you hit your local fast-food drive-thru a few times a week or are used to (we'd even say hooked on) eating refined carbohydrates and sugars every day, you might want to ease into things. People fail at making dietary changes for several reasons, but one we'd like you to check at the door is catastrophizing, or all-or-nothing thinking.

Moving in the right direction, even generally, is progress. Period. You can't ruin a diet or your health with a single meal or fast-food binge. The best way to keep smiling is to keep trying.

During an investigation of a price-fixing scheme, an officer of Archer Daniels Midland, one of America's largest food processors, was quoted as stating, "We have a saying at this company—our competitors are our friends and our customers are our enemies."

Try incorporating one or two meal plans a week, ideally the seafood meals. If you don't eat much seafood yet, maybe start with something more familiar, like one of our pork dishes.

But just like quitting smoking, a lot of people decide to go cold turkey—and if that's your method, we've got you covered for two weeks. Either way, it's time to get started.

The Happiness Diet Meal Plan—
Week One

Day 1

Breakfast

1 small container whole-milk plain Greek yogurt
1 handful raspberries or blueberries
1 teaspoon maple syrup (to sweeten yogurt, if needed)
Splash of whole milk or half-and-half (optional)

Lunch

Middle Eastern Picnic:
- 1 cup Humble Hummus (page 175)
- 1 cup Barley Tabbouleh (page 184)
- 1 chunk feta cheese (the size of a deck of cards)
- 1 cup oil-cured olives
- 1 whole wheat pita

Snack

Almond Butter Ants on a Log:
- 2 celery sticks
- 2 tablespoons almond butter
- Handful organic raisins

Spread almond butter into celery groove. Add raisins on top. Kids like this one.

Dinner

Steamed Mussels (or Clams) (page 204)
2 tablespoons melted butter with lemon juice, for dipping
Ginger Green Beans (page 183)

TOP 100 REASONS TO AVOID PROCESSED FOODS

Eating processed food contributes to the death of small farms across America.

Day ②

Hard-Boiled Egg Breakfast (page 168)
½ grapefruit, topped with ½ teaspoon honey

Lunch
Happy Fish Salad Sandwich (page 210)
Simple Salad (page 186)

Snack
2–3 slivers of cheese
1 apple (organic)

Dinner
Butter Lettuce Salad (page 192)
Roasted Chicken and Vegetables (page 195)
Prepare to Smile: Do a quick prep for breakfast tomorrow by soaking oatmeal in milk overnight in fridge.

Day ③

Breakfast
1 cup Almond Joy Oats (page 166)
Splash of whole milk or half-and-half (optional)

Lunch
Chicken Salad Sandwich (page 208)

Snack
1 handful almonds
1 apple (organic)

Dinner
The HD Burger (page 200)
2 cups kale sautéed in butter and dressed in a vinaigrette
1 ear of corn, with butter

Day 4

Breakfast

Mexican Breakfast (page 170)

Lunch

Tomato-Basil Soup (page 178)
Brussels Sprouts with Bacon (page 185)

Snack

Carrot sticks and hummus

Dinner

Simple Salad (page 186)
Happy Wild Salmon (page 212)
Roasted Cauliflower (page 180)

Day 5

Breakfast

Perfectly Scrambled Eggs (page 165)

Lunch

Happy Fish Salad Sandwiches (page 210)

Snack

Pepitas (pumpkin seeds)
1 orange

Dinner

Belgian Endive Salad (page 193)
Perfect Pork Chops (page 209)

TOP 100 REASONS TO AVOID PROCESSED FOODS

Milk from factory-farmed cows treated with growth hormone often
contains pus.

Day

Breakfast
Smiling Swedish Breakfast (page 169)

Lunch
The Happiness Diet EBLT (page 211)
1 pear (organic)

Snack
1 small handful walnuts
1 small handful cacao nibs

Dinner
Grass-Fed Balsamic Flank Steak (page 213)
Rocket Salad (page 000)
Roasted Mushrooms (page 174)

Day

Breakfast
Old-Fashioned Bacon and Eggs (page 171)

Lunch
Steak Salad:
Arugula with leftover steak and vinaigrette (page 218)

Snack
Cashews

Dinner
Raw Brussels Sprout Salad (page 194)
Oven-Roasted Cod (page 206)
Smashed Purple Potatoes (page 176)

TOP 100 REASONS TO AVOID PROCESSED FOODS

Just because jelly bean and soda manufacturers tout antioxidants in
their products doesn't mean their food is healthful.

The Happiness Diet Meal Plan—
Week Two

The Happiness Diet isn't progressive. You can mix and match anything from the first week into the second week and vice versa. The weeks as presented here are to give you a clearer picture of the options you have available when choosing "happy" foods. Remember, these menus are here to help, not overwhelm. If preparing all of the meals in the plans seems too much for you right now, try to make a rule of substituting one meal in your diet each day. Then add another and another until these foods are what you and your body are thriving on. Start wherever you can and just keep building. This week we toss in a vegetarian day, our nod to the Meatless Monday movement. This simple adjustment drastically drops your environmental impact.

Day

Breakfast
Perfectly Scrambled Eggs (page 165)

Lunch
Butternut Squash Soup (page 177)
Rocket Salad (page 172)
Kale-Octopus Bites (page 188)

Snack
Raw almonds

Dinner
Grass-Fed Meatballs Marinara (page 202)
Zucchini Carpaccio (page 187)

Day 2

Breakfast

1 container whole-milk plain Greek yogurt with 1 handful raspberries or blueberries and ¼ teaspoon cinnamon

Lunch

Beans and Rice (page 181)

Snack

1 handful unsalted pistachio nuts
4–5 grape or cherry tomatoes

Dinner

Simple Salad (page 186)
Roasted Cauliflower (page 180)
Cream of Tomato Soup (page 179)

Day 3

Breakfast

Old-Fashioned Bacon and Eggs (page 171)

Lunch

Tuna over Greens (page 199)

Snack

½ avocado topped with juice from 1 wedge of lemon

Dinner

Perfect Pork Chops (page 209)
Broccoli with Anchovies (page 173)

TOP 100 REASONS TO AVOID PROCESSED FOODS

The National Pork Board (industrial pig farmers) is so fearful of the rising popularity of naturally raised pigs that they funded a study to show that pasture-raised pork has higher rates of salmonella, toxoplasma, and trichina than pigs reared in factory farms. Scary news, if true, but they misrepresented their findings. All the researchers found was more antibodies in the natural pigs for those diseases. Which is to say that the study simply showed that pasture-raised pigs have better immune systems.

Day

Breakfast
Whole wheat toast topped with almond or peanut butter and banana slices, drizzled with honey

Lunch
Citrus Spinach Salad (page 182)
1 small button of goat cheese with brown rice crackers

Snack
2–3 slices hard salami
2–3 pieces of your favorite cheese

Dinner
Simple Salad (page 186)
Ginger Mackerel (page 205)
Roasted Cauliflower (page 180)

Day 5

Breakfast
Perfectly Scrambled Eggs (page 165)

Lunch
Mexican Squid (page 197)

Snack
Kale chips

Dinner
Ginger-Beet Soup (page 189)
Flawless Grilled Chicken (page 207)

TOP 100 REASONS TO AVOID PROCESSED FOODS

Tyson had to pay a $5.2 million fine for bribing two veterinarians at Mexico's agriculture department to not create problems at a plant that processed chicken into stuff like patties and chicken tenders. The company had previously been accused of trying to bribe the US Secretary of Agriculture.

Day 6

Breakfast

Hard-Boiled Egg Breakfast (page 168)

Lunch

½ avocado

4–5 cherry tomatoes, halved

1–2 pieces leftover Flawless Grilled Chicken

Snack

Fresh fruit with kefir or yogurt

Dinner

Spicy Fish Stew (page 214)

Simple Salad (page 186)

Day 7

Breakfast

Oatmeal with walnuts, berries, and cream

Lunch

Fish tacos using leftovers from Day 5's dinner

Snack

Carrots, broccoli, and cauliflower, sprinkled with ½ teaspoon of crumbled blue cheese

Dinner

Simple Salad (page 186)

Slow Pork (page 198)

Braised Red Cabbage Salad (page 191)

TOP 100 REASONS TO AVOID PROCESSED FOODS

Candy Dynamics recently recalled all flavors of its "Toxic Waste" brand "Nuclear Sludge" chew bars because of elevated levels of the neurotoxin lead.

Happiness on the Run: What to Eat at the Office, Gym, or Local Restaurants

At the Office

Anxious eating happens most often at work. Instead of patronizing the vending machine or dipping into cake and soda from the office party, fill your desk drawers with snacks that grow your brain. You will improve your performance . . . and cut down on the stress.

Store in your desk:

- Green tea bags
- Whole unsalted almonds
- Cacao nibs (nature's Red Bull)
- Fresh fruit
- Hard salami
- Miniature dark chocolate bars (we crave a sweet sometimes, and studies show these can improve focus for two to three hours)
- Kale chips (the ultimate potato chip alternative)
- Cheese

If Work Has You Lunching Out

- If fast food is all that's available, pick an establishment like Chipotle that gives you high-quality natural meat that you can eat over greens.

TOP 100 REASONS TO AVOID PROCESSED FOODS

No matter what the packaging says: Processed foods are made to be cheap—not healthy.

- Skip the deli meats at sandwich shops and instead load up on veggies. Grab a veggie and cheese sandwich from Subway. Go easy on the bread.
- Enjoy sushi but go easy on the rice, and pick brown rice if it is available. If not, remove some of the white rice from a few of the sushi pieces.

At the Gym

This one is simple: Pack up some food rather than packing it in and not hitting the gym. Here are a few ideas:

- Bananas
- Hard-cooked eggs
- Hummus and veggies
- Leftover meatballs
- Nuts
- Whole-milk yogurt

Nights Out

Some of the same tips for lunching will apply here if you're just going out for something casual. But if you're making a real night of it, keep these pointers in mind and you'll stay on the right path:

TOP 100 REASONS TO AVOID PROCESSED FOODS

Bisphenol A (BPA), a chemical found in many canned foods and bottled waters, damages brain synapses, resulting in an increased risk of depression and impaired memory.

- Find anything on the menu that is local or wild.
- Try to avoid bread, pizza, and pasta.
- Always start with a salad and get the dressing on the side or ask for oil and vinegar. Or go with soup, if you prefer.
- Pile your plate with vegetables whether you order the salad or not.
- Split dessert or skip it (you'll know if you've had too much sugar that day/week or if you can splurge).

TOP 100 REASONS TO AVOID PROCESSED FOODS

Many artificial food colorings are synthesized from coal tar and are linked to attention deficit hyperactivity disorder (ADHD), according to research published in the journal *Lancet*.

9

Our Favorite Recipes

We often hear that our brain is Mother Nature's most complex creation. But there's something even more enigmatic, paradoxical, and sophisticated than the gray matter that fills the space between our ears: the food chain that evolved over millions of years to provide fuel for our brains. We're omnivores by nature and, as such, we rely on a complex set of nutrients from minerals, plants, and animals for optimal health. But eating was never meant to be fussy or complicated.

It wasn't so long ago that rural America mirrored the "epicurean" lifestyle of Tuscany and Provence that we seek to emulate today. Recipes and the know-how of food preparation were based on family traditions, passed down from mother to daughter for generations. It wasn't until 1796, when an orphan by the name of Amelia Simmons decided to educate single women on the basics of cooking, that the first American cookbook came into existence: *American Cookery*. Simmons fought her editor's suggestion to include material about choosing meat and vegetables at the market because she thought it was insulting to suggest that women wouldn't have these basic skills.

Within a hundred years, however, this knowledge disappeared, and food marketing filled the vacuum. Along the way, a lot of us lost the simple, intuitive knowledge of "cookery." Eventually, in 1936, widowed homemaker Irma S. Rombauer published what would become the bible of the American kitchen: *The Joy of Cooking.* The first cookbook to include precise measurements and instructions, it has been a powerful influence on the way we think about food preparation, including the common perception that making meals at home is a chore.

In the pages that follow, you won't find any recipes that require laser-like precision. These meals are designed around the idea of using nature's own mood boosters to create delicious, simple dishes that allow plenty of room for improvisation so that you can develop your own cookery skills.

TOP 100 REASONS TO AVOID PROCESSED FOODS

Interesterified fats, the new industrial fats replacing trans fats, are virtually unstudied for their long-term health effects, but emerging data give reason for concern.

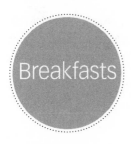

Breakfasts

Perfectly Scrambled Eggs

Scrambled eggs can be endlessly tweaked with a little intuitiveness. There are only a few guiding principles to follow. Always add cheese, but not too much, and make sure it's grated. Add more black pepper than you think is reasonable. And if you're adding any kind of vegetables (say, leftover brussels sprouts), make sure you cook the produce first and then add the eggs, cheese, and seasoning last.

Eggs are not just for breakfast. They can be eaten any mealtime. They're brain food. They're high in choline, the precursor of the neurotransmitter acetylcholine, which is key for our energy, focus, and memory. They are packed with omega-3s and vitamin B_{12}, both of which are used to treat depression. And when you mix them with garlic and olive oil, you add a variety of phytochemicals and antioxidants known to support good vascular health and stave off common causes of depression and dementia later in life.

- 2 **eggs**
- 1 **tablespoon butter**
- 2 **cloves garlic, minced**
   Salt and freshly ground black pepper
- 2 **ounces blue cheese, Manchego, or Gouda (grated)**

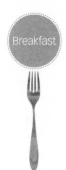

MAKE IT: Crack the eggs into a bowl; whisk together and set aside. Melt the butter in a skillet over medium heat; add the garlic and cook until fragrant. Pour the eggs into the skillet, stirring occasionally, and add salt and pepper to taste. Add the cheese after a few minutes, spreading evenly over the mixture. When the cheese is just melted, remove the eggs from the pan and serve immediately.

(Serves 1)

Almond Joy Oats

These oats are softened overnight in milk, covered and stored in your fridge. As they cook in the morning, you may catch a whiff of the tropics from the coconut oil. Just be sure to go easy on the cacao nibs, as too many can get you overly revved up. Oats are very high in tryptophan and selenium, two nutrients known to affect mood. Almonds get your morning started with lots of alpha-tocotrienol, a form of vitamin E being investigated for its neuroprotective properties.

This recipe is dedicated to our agent, Joy.

1	**cup steel-cut oats**
2	**cups whole milk**
1	**teaspoon coconut oil**
1	**teaspoon cacao nibs**
¹⁄₂	**cup organic shaved coconut**
¹⁄₂	**cup almonds, chopped**

MAKE IT: Mix the oats and milk together in a bowl. Cover and refrigerate overnight. In the morning, warm the coconut oil and nibs over low heat. Then top with shaved coconut and almonds and enjoy.

(Serves 2)

Lemon Yogurt–Topped Fresh Fruit

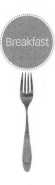

This simple, quick breakfast or snack is a great source of energy and nutrients. Flavoring it yourself with fresh lemon and a little bit of molasses means you can steer clear of the artificial sweeteners, colorings, and flavors in many commercially available yogurts. Spoon this lemony yogurt over a bowl of fresh berries, melon, or whatever fruit is in season. The more colors in your bowl, the more varieties of brain-protecting phytonutrients like anthocyanins and lycopene. A little molasses fortifies this dish with iron and magnesium. Fresh lemon zest is loaded with flavonoids that reduce brain inflammation.

1 **lemon**

1 **cup cream-top yogurt**

1 **tablespoon blackstrap molasses**

Kosher or sea salt

Fresh fruit (dependent on season)

MAKE IT: Zest a few tablespoons of lemon peel and stir into the yogurt. Slice the lemon in half and use a citrus squeezer to juice half of the lemon into the yogurt. Mix in the molasses and add a pinch of salt to taste. Spoon over a bowl of fresh fruit.

(Serves 2)

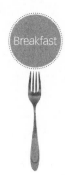

Hard-Boiled Egg Breakfast

As we've shown you, eggs are a perfect brain food. They're loaded with fats that will keep you full and thinking sharply. The list of brain-healthy essential elements of happiness that are contained in eggs is off the charts: B_{12}, vitamin D, omega-3s, iodine, magnesium, and on and on. This quick, simple breakfast can also be served as a side at dinner.

2 **eggs**

2 **scallions, chopped**

1 **lemon**

Salt and freshly ground black pepper

1 **tablespoon olive oil**

MAKE IT: Put the eggs in water in a saucepan over medium heat. When the water begins to boil, turn the heat to low. Cook the eggs for 10 to 15 minutes; drain. Use a sharp knife or an egg slicer to cut the eggs into thin strips. Lay on a plate and sprinkle with scallions, zest from the lemon, and salt and pepper to taste. Drizzle with the olive oil and enjoy.

(Serves 1)

TOP 100 REASONS TO AVOID PROCESSED FOODS

Cockroaches and flies that visit factory farms are becoming resistant to antibiotics, and researchers at North Carolina State University fear these bugs may spread this resistance into nearby towns.

Smiling Swedish Breakfast

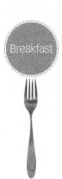

Getting enough omega-3s is key for optimal brain health. Eating salmon for breakfast is a great way to start, as it's packed with DHA and EPA. Flaxseed bread is also particularly high in omega-3s. You can also find other dense, dark breads made with sunflower seeds and nuts. Higher in fiber than regular varieties, these breads don't lead to spikes in blood sugar and give you the added benefit of more minerals like nerve-soothing magnesium and a variety of phytonutrients.

2	tablespoons whole-milk (full-fat) cream cheese
2	pieces flaxseed bread
2	ounces wild smoked salmon or trout
	Handful of capers
	Sliced red onion, diced
1–2	teaspoons of red wine vinegar
1	tablespoon olive oil
	Salt and freshly ground black pepper
2	cups strawberries

MAKE IT: Spread the cream cheese, evenly divided, on each slice of bread. Top with the fish. Sprinkle the capers and onion over the fish. Next, mix the vinegar and olive oil in a bowl and then drizzle over the salmon. Add salt and pepper to taste. Serve with the strawberries.

(Serves 1)

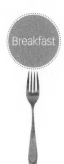

Breakfast

Mexican Breakfast

Instead of pairing eggs with a breakfast meat for your morning protein, look to beans to provide a plethora of nutrients. They are an amazing source of folate, fiber, magnesium, and iron—which by now you know are key to brain health. Beans also contain important starches that are vital for gut health and a variety of brain-protecting phytonutrients like anthocyanins and quercetin. Adding avocado's great mix of fats means better absorption of nutrients like the lycopene and beta-carotene found in the salsa. Warmed corn tortillas make this an easy, quick breakfast to go.

1 teaspoon lard (or butter)

1 cup beans

3 eggs

4 corn tortillas (check label for ingredients first and buy
   one with corn and lard . . . and no unpronounceables)

1 avocado, peeled and sliced

1 lime, juiced
   Dash of cayenne pepper

2 tablespoons grated Cheddar cheese

2 tablespoons salsa

MAKE IT: Melt the lard in a skillet over medium heat. Add the beans. In a separate bowl, crack and whisk the eggs. Warm the tortillas in a toaster oven or covered in a microwave for 15 seconds. Move the beans to one side of the skillet, or remove them and set aside. In a small bowl, mash the avocado, lime juice, and cayenne pepper together with a fork; set aside. Pour the eggs into the skillet and scramble. Fill the tortillas with a layer of beans, eggs, grated cheese, and avocado; top with salsa.

(Serves 2)

Old-Fashioned Bacon and Eggs

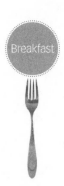

We've told you about the brain benefits of eating more eggs. Now let's slip some more brain-essential nutrients into your diet with bacon. Pasture-raised pigs contain vitamin D, and the main fat in bacon, oleic acid, is linked to a decreased risk of depression in women. Both bacon and eggs contain choline, which is linked to lower anxiety, and CLA, which reduces belly fat and fights cancer.

- 2   **strips bacon**
- 2   **eggs**
    Salt and freshly ground black pepper
- 1   **cup coffee**

MAKE IT: In a large skillet, cook the bacon for 5 minutes over low heat. Flip with tongs and cook until the bacon is just crispy. Set aside. Crack the eggs into the pan. Cook until the yolks are firm. Add salt and pepper to taste. Enjoy with a cup of coffee.

(Serves 1)

TOP 100 REASONS TO AVOID PROCESSED FOODS

So many people are getting fat in developing nations as the MAD diet spreads that scientists have developed the term "fat cancers" for cancers like that of the breast and colon that are associated with being overweight.

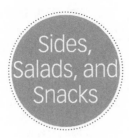

Sides, Salads, and Snacks

Rocket Salad

As a member of the cruciferous family, arugula is packed with disease-fighting sulfur compounds like glucosinolates. These compounds get diminished when heated, so eating them raw in a salad is a great choice. Arugula is also higher in calcium, iron, folate, and beta-carotene than other greens. Adding some Parmesan cheese, walnuts, and olive oil ensures the proper digestion and absorption of key fat-soluble nutrients, like vitamin K, that keep your blood running smoothly. Walnuts also add a dose of the omega-3 fat ALA, fat-protecting vitamin E, and a bevy of antioxidants that defend the brain from free radicals.

  1   **pound arugula**
      Parmesan cheese
$^1/_2$ **cup chopped walnuts**
      Olive oil
      Red wine vinegar
      Balsamic vinegar
      Salt and freshly ground black pepper

MAKE IT: Wash and dry the arugula and then top with generous portion of freshly grated Parmesan cheese and the walnuts. In a small bowl, mix a few tablespoons of olive oil with red wine vinegar and a dash of balsamic vinegar. Add salt and pepper to taste. Spoon the vinaigrette over the salad and enjoy.

(Serves 2)

Broccoli with Anchovies

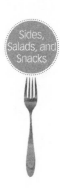

You'll notice the use of ice baths in this chapter, and that's because vegetables don't stop cooking just because you've pulled them off the stove. This is where the ice bath comes in. Dunking the broccoli in ice water immediately stops the vegetable from cooking so you can ensure a perfect texture each time. Broccoli is packed with isothiocyanates—molecules that activate our most potent cancer-fighting pathways. It also has more vitamin C than an orange. To make it taste good, you need not only the right texture but also a proper dressing. We recommend one with anchovies. It's a savory mixture that beats back the blues with omega-3s, vitamin D, and lots of B-complex vitamins. As you'll see, it's a great dressing—one you can use on most vegetables.

- 1 **can anchovies in olive oil**
- 3 **tablespoons olive oil**
- 1 **lemon**
- ½ **chile pepper, minced (wear plastic gloves when handling)**
- 2 **garlic cloves, minced**
  Salt and freshly ground black pepper
- 2 **pounds broccoli, trimmed**

MAKE IT: Drain the anchovies and soak in water for 5 to 10 minutes to remove excess salt. Drain and place in a medium-size bowl. Add the olive oil, juice of the lemon, chile pepper, and garlic. Mash and add salt and pepper to taste. Set aside. Boil water with 1 tablespoon of salt in a 3-quart pot. In a large bowl, prepare an ice bath by filling it three-quarters full with cold water and ice cubes. Add the broccoli florets to boiling water and cook for 3 to 5 minutes, depending on the size of the florets, or until bright green and just starting to soften. Remove the broccoli with a strainer and immediately place in the ice bath for 1 minute. Florets should be tender yet slightly crisp. Drain the broccoli and place in a large bowl. Toss with the dressing and serve.

(Serves 4)

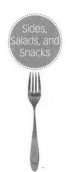

Roasted Mushrooms

Mushrooms expose us to a variety of unique health-promoting molecules. Lentinan, for example, is an immune booster and anti-cancer agent that is used in cancer chemotherapy. Lovastatin, another natural compound, is synthesized by drug manufacturers to regulate cholesterol. Mushrooms are also great sources of trace minerals like copper, which is essential for collagen production and healthy skin.

1 **pound oyster or shiitake mushrooms**

4 **tablespoons olive oil**

3–5 **sprigs fresh thyme**

Salt and freshly ground black pepper

3 **tablespoons butter**

MAKE IT: Preheat the oven to 325 degrees. Rinse the mushrooms and break apart either with your hands (in the case of oysters) or with a knife (in the case of shiitakes). Discard and tough stems. Coat a small baking dish with some of the olive oil. Spread the mushrooms evenly along the bottom of the dish. Remove the leaves from the sprigs of thyme and sprinkle them over the mushrooms. Salt and pepper liberally. Slice off four thin tabs of butter and place around the dish on top of the mushrooms. Drizzle 2 tablespoons of olive oil over the mix and cook for 30 minutes.

(Serves 4)

Humble Hummus

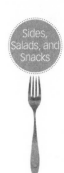

Sides, Salads, and Snacks

This dish will get your motor running so you can power through the afternoon on a smooth ride of complete protein from legumes. We swap out the traditional chickpeas for red beans and you are consuming nature's antioxidant champion. Once you nail the below recipe, experiment with spices like basil or dill to keep this dish fun and interesting.

- 1   **can chickpeas or red beans**
- 1   **clove garlic**
- 1   **tablespoon olive oil**
- 1   **tablespoon lemon peel**

MAKE IT: Rinse beans in a colander under cold water. Place all the ingredients in a small food processor or blender. Mix for about 1 minute, or until creamy. Serve on fresh cucumber slices or your favorite crudité.

(Serves 4)

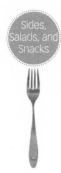

Smashed Purple Potatoes

We most commonly encounter potatoes in the MAD as french fries and potato chips. Potato chips were the food most clearly linked to obesity in a large study by Harvard Medical School. But small colored potatoes are loaded with nutrients. Keep the skin on to ensure you get these spuds' full dose of iron, folate, fiber, and B_6. One medium potato contains twice as much vitamin C as a tomato, and potatoes are a good source of iodine needed for a healthy thyroid gland. A stellar set of phytonutrients includes kukoamines that lower blood pressure and chlorogenic acid, a powerful antioxidant that helps regulate blood sugar. We add grass-fed butter for some belly-reducing CLA.

- 8   **medium purple potatoes**
- 1   **cup whole milk**
- 2   **tablespoons butter**
  Salt and freshly ground black pepper

MAKE IT: Scrub any dirt from the potatoes, then boil them for 20 minutes. Briefly rinse with cold water. Smash with a fork. Mix in milk, butter, and salt and pepper to taste.

(Serves 4)

Butternut Squash Soup

This is a classic of late summer and early fall, and it's great for freezing to eat all year long. Surprising to some, squash has about a third of the omega-3s as walnuts. But it's also loaded with vitamin C and carotenoids—antioxidants that fight inflammation and protect against all the diseases of the MAD way of life.

1	large butternut squash
1–2	tablespoons fresh ginger, peeled and finely diced
5	small leeks (white part only; the smaller ones have more flavor than the large)
$1/_2$	stick butter or 4 tablespoons olive oil (or a mixture of both)
3–4	cups chicken stock, depending on consistency preference
	Salt and freshly ground black pepper

MAKE IT: Preheat the oven to 400 degrees. Take the squash and cut it in half lengthwise. Scoop out the seeds (they can be saved and used as a garnish). Place the squash cut side down on a baking sheet and bake for 45 to 60 minutes, depending on the size of the squash, until a knife easily pierces the flesh. About 15 minutes before the squash comes out of the oven, place a pot on the stove, add the butter/olive oil, and melt over medium heat. Place the ginger and leeks in the melted butter and cook for about 10 minutes on medium heat until soft—do not let it brown. Scoop the squash out of its skin and add to the pot. Pour in the chicken stock and bring to a simmer. Let simmer for 30 to 60 minutes. (The longer it reduces, the better; more stock can be added later for those who like thinner soup). Blend the soup in a food processor or blender and add salt and pepper to taste.

(Serves 2)

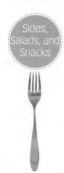

Tomato-Basil Soup

This soup is excellent warm or cold and has deep flavor thanks to its reliance on a handful of different types of tomatoes. Top it with crème fraîche for a contrast of flavors that deepens the savory roasted flavor of the tomatoes. The combination of pepper, garlic, and onions fights inflammation and all the diseases—from depression to cancer—associated with it. It also freezes well.

> **Roughly 8 tomatoes (preferably a mixture of plum, heirloom, or whatever is in season), quartered or halved, depending on size**
>
> 1 **carton cherry tomatoes**
>
> **Olive oil and/or butter**
>
> **Salt and freshly ground black pepper**
>
> 1 **clove garlic, minced**
>
> 2 **small yellow onions, chopped**
>
> 1 **cup chopped sweet onions**
>
> 1 **teaspoon crushed red pepper flakes (more or less depending on penchant)**
>
> 1 **cup coarsely chopped fresh basil, stems removed**
>
> 1 **cup San Marzano crushed tomatoes**
>
> 3–4 **cups chicken stock**

MAKE IT: Preheat the oven to 375 degrees. Toss the tomatoes with a liberal amount of olive oil and salt and pepper. Put in cast iron pan and bake for 30 to 40 minutes.

In large pot, add 2 to 3 tablespoons olive oil or butter and cook the garlic, onions, and red pepper flakes, making sure none of it browns. Add the tomatoes from the oven and pour in all the juices from the pan. Add the basil and San Marzano tomatoes. Add the chicken stock and let simmer (nearly boil) for an hour. Blend until smooth. More stock can be added if a thinner consistency is preferred.

(Serves 4)

Cream of Tomato Soup

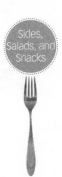

You can make a cream soup out of nearly any vegetable. Here is the classic for a great after-school snack or ski house staple. You'll prep this in minutes and reap the benefits of eating foods with lycopene for life.

6	**large tomatoes**
1	**medium onion**
2	**tablespoons olive oil**
2	**cloves garlic, minced**
4	**cups water or vegetable stock**
1	**pint half-and-half (to desired thickness)**
½	**cup chopped fresh basil**
	Salt and freshly ground black pepper

MAKE IT: Chop the tomatoes and onion coarsely. In a large pot, add the olive oil and garlic. Cook over medium heat for a few minutes, then add the tomatoes and onion. After 10 minutes, add the water or vegetable stock. Simmer for 30 minutes. Stir in the half-and-half and basil. Simmer for 15 minutes and add salt and pepper to taste. Serve.

(Serves 4)

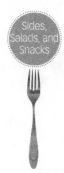

Roasted Cauliflower

Cauliflower is very high in vitamin C and fiber and loaded with vitamin B$_6$ and folate, both important cofactors needed for the production of several key neurotransmitters. Inadequate levels of these nutrients are linked to low mood, low energy, and dementia. Eating just one serving a day of vegetables like cauliflower has been shown to decrease the chance of developing the most aggressive forms of prostate cancer.

1 **large head cauliflower**
3 **tablespoons olive oil**
2 **lemons**
   Salt and freshly ground black pepper
3 **tablespoons butter**

MAKE IT: Preheat the oven to 400 degrees. Break the cauliflower into bite-size florets and place in a baking dish. Drizzle with the olive oil. Squeeze the juice of 1½ lemons over the cauliflower. Season liberally with salt and pepper. Cut the butter into slivers and place around the baking dish. Roast for 45 minutes, or until the cauliflower is lightly browned. Remove the dish from the oven, squeeze the remaining lemon half over the cauliflower, and serve.

(Serves 4)

94

TOP 100 REASONS TO AVOID PROCESSED FOODS

Those blueberries found in cereal, muffins, and bagels? They're often fake. Made of nothing more than sugar, hydrogenated oil, and artificial food dyes No. 2 and No. 40.

Beans and Rice

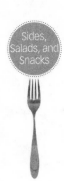

By combining rice and beans, you get all the essential amino acids you need to build proteins, and that's one of the reasons this combo is such a popular staple around the world. Swap out white or instant rice for a whole grain like basmati or brown rice and you'll get the benefit of slowly digestible starches, minerals like magnesium, and one of the top sources of brain-protecting toco-trienols, rice bran. Studies show that the rice-and-bean synergy extend to vitamin E, which increases by sixteen times when you add black beans. Or pick red beans for the winner of the most antioxidant power, according to studies by the USDA.

2	**cups dried beans, or 2 (12-ounce) cans beans**
1	**cup rice**
	Salt and freshly ground black pepper
	Olive oil
2	**medium yellow onions, chopped**
1	**organic red bell pepper, chopped**
	Chili powder or fresh chile peppers
1/4	**pound Cheddar cheese, sliced**

MAKE IT: If using dried beans, cover them in water in a large pot and bring to a boil. Reduce to simmer for 2 hours, cover, and add water as needed. If using canned beans, simply rinse and set aside. In another covered pot, make the rice according to the package instructions. In a skillet, combine a few tablespoons of olive oil with the onions and peppers and cook until the the onions become translucent. Add to beans and stir. Add salt, pepper, and chili powder or chile peppers to taste. Scoop the rice over the beans and top with cheese.

(Serves 4)

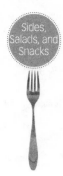

Citrus Spinach Salad

This salad is packed with our favorite brain-saving phytonutrients: ellagatannins, anthocyanins, tocotrienols, and folates, to name a few. Walnuts have a near-perfect 1 to 3 ratio of omega-3 to omega-6 fatty acids along with a nerve-calming dose of magnesium. The sweet, tangy crunch of the pomegranate seeds contains massive amounts of ellagitannins, one of nature's most powerful antioxidants.

1	**orange**
1	**pomegranate**
2	**bunches spinach**
2	**tablespoons olive oil**
$\frac{1}{2}$	**cup pine nuts**
	Salt

MAKE IT: Zest and then juice half of the orange. Cut the pomegranate into quarters and collect the fruit. Rinse the spinach in cold water. Spread the spinach on a clean kitchen towel, then roll the spinach in the towel to dry it. Mix the orange zest, juice, olive oil, and pine nuts together. Add salt to taste. Thirty minutes prior to serving, mix the spinach and dressing. Add the pomegranate fruit.

(Serves 4)

Ginger Green Beans

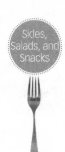

Bring your green beans to the next level with this simple recipe that will have your family clamoring for more. Which is important, because green beans are packed with fiber, folate, vitamin K, vitamin A, and vitamin C. Ginger contains compounds that combat the damage from the sun's UVB rays, fight nausea, lower stress, and fight inflammation. And this recipe is a failure-proof side that pairs well with everything from fish to pork chops to steak.

1 **pound green beans**

3 **tablespoons butter**

4 **cloves garlic, minced**

4 **ounces fresh ginger, shredded or chopped**

2 **medium vine-ripe tomatoes, chopped**

3 **tablespoons olive oil**

   Salt and freshly ground black pepper

MAKE IT: Rinse the green beans, trim the tips, and set aside. Melt the butter in a 2-quart pan over medium heat. Add the garlic and ginger and cook for 1 or 2 minutes. Add the green beans, tomatoes, and olive oil and cover, reducing the heat slightly. Stir frequently and season to taste with salt and pepper. Remove from heat after 7 to 10 minutes; the green beans should still be somewhat crisp. Transfer the beans to a serving bowl and top with the leftover sauce.

(Serves 4)

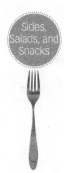

Barley Tabbouleh

Use barley to make a hearty lunch and to get all eight forms of tocopherols and tocotrienols, also known as vitamin E. This whole grain contains beta-glucan, a form of fiber that improves insulin resistance, and the parsley provides ample folates and fiber. Lemon zest supercharges this dish with citrus phytonutrients like liminoids.

- 1 **cup dry barley**
- 1 **small bunch parsley**
- 1 **cup diced cherry tomatoes**
- 1 **small cucumber, chopped**
- 2 **tablespoons olive oil**
  Zest and juice from ½ lemon

MAKE IT: Place the barley and 2 cups water in a covered pot and bring to a boil, then reduce the heat and simmer for 25 minutes. When the water is absorbed, place the barley in a bowl in the refrigerator and chill. Meanwhile, chop the parsley. Mix the cherry tomatoes, cucumbers, olive oil, and lemon zest and juice in a bowl. Combine the barley, vegetables, and chopped parsley shortly before serving.

(Serves 2)

Brussels Sprouts with Bacon

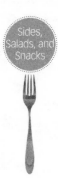

When you're preparing brussels sprouts, try to loosen up the leaves a little with your hands so they soften and fall apart a bit as they cook. Mixing a little butter with the olive oil in this recipe prevents oxidation, which can damage the fats and make them unhealthy. These fats also make the vitamin K in the sprouts more available to the body. Keep in mind that brussels sprouts are just like scrambled eggs in that they can be endlessly tweaked depending on your mood. Try adding cheese or roasted nuts and you'll be pleasantly surprised with your results.

24   brussels sprouts
 3   tablespoons extra virgin olive oil
 2   tablespoons butter
 4   cloves garlic, diced
 1   yellow onion, chopped
 4   strips cooked bacon
     Salt and freshly ground black pepper

MAKE IT: Rinse the brussels sprouts under cool water and remove any tough or damaged outer leaves. Trim the stems and cut the sprouts into quarters. Set aside. Add the olive oil and butter to a deep-sided skillet and place over medium-high heat. Add the garlic and cook for 1 or 2 minutes, until fragrant. Add the onion and cook for 5 minutes, or until translucent. Add the brussels sprouts and bacon and cover; cook for about 17 minutes, or until the sprouts are just soft. Don't overcook your sprouts; they will continue to cook once you've removed them from the pan because their fibrous bodies retain heat. Be gentle with them, as well: the less you stir, the more the sugars will caramelize and the vegetable will take on a nutty, sweet flavor.

(Serves 4)

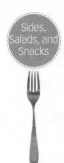

Simple Salad

Putting more vegetables on your plate is a pillar of the Happiness Diet, and the variations of salads are nearly endless. Or you can just keep it simple. Mesclun is our top focus food, as you get plenty of folate that helps preserve your cognitive abilities and prevent depression. The mix of leaves in mesclun gives you a wide variety of phytonutrients like carotenoids that promote health and happiness. Onions are surprisingly concentrated with powerful phytonutrients like quercetin and the mineral chromium, which is linked to mood and insulin function.

2 **cups washed mesclun**
¼ **cup thinly sliced red onion**
1 **tablespoon grated Parmesan**
5 **cherry tomatoes, halved**
2 **tablespoons vinaigrette dressing (see page 218)**

MAKE IT: Place all the ingredients together in a big salad or mixing bowl; gently toss for about a minute, until the veggies are well-dressed. Enjoy now, as dressed lettuces wilt in the fridge and just don't taste very good.

(Serves 1 as a meal, 2 as a side)

TOP 100 REASONS TO AVOID PROCESSED FOODS

Taco Bell has been sued for false advertising for referring to its meat mixture as "beef." The complaint stated that the company has so many binders and extenders in the product that it doesn't meet the minimum requirements of the USDA to be labeled as "beef."

Zucchini Carpaccio

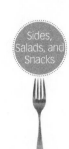

This playful take on beef carpaccio is surprisingly addictive—and seriously healthy. Zucchini is loaded with folate, which fights depression and decreases your blood level of homocysteine—a reliable marker for heart disease and decreased brain function. Mint settles the stomach and has antibacterial properties known to kill foodborne toxins like *E. coli*. Parmesan cheese ensures you extract all the fat-soluble antioxidants from the greens to protect your brain and heart from free radicals.

2   medium zucchini
1   leek
    Salt and freshly ground black pepper
1   tablespoon extra virgin olive oil
1   lemon, juiced
    Fresh chunk of Parmesan
    Handful of fresh mint leaves, cut into slivers

MAKE IT: Use a mandoline to slice the zucchini and leek into very thin rounds (a sharp knife will also work). Overlap the zucchini disks on a plate. Season with salt and pepper to taste. Drizzle with the olive oil and lemon juice. Sprinkle with the sliced leeks. Using your mandoline or a cheese slicer, shave very thin slices of Parmesan to spread over the leeks. Garnish with the mint and serve.

(Serves 4)

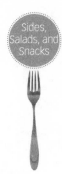
Kale-Octopus Bites

Octopus is a rarely eaten power food, and you can find a nice canned version in the Asian section of your grocery store or at Asian specialty markets. (You can substitute smoked fish in a pinch.) Octopus is high in omega-3s, B_{12}, B_6, iron, and selenium. All these nutrients play a role in making neurotransmitters. Octopus also contains large amounts of taurine, an amino acid that relaxes your mind and body. Combining it with sardines and kale adds even more omega-3s, folate, and fiber for a snack that fights diseases.

- 1 **head kale**
- 1 **can anchovies**
- 3 **tablespoons olive oil**
- 1 **lemon, juiced**
- 2 **cloves garlic, minced**
     Salt and freshly ground black pepper
- 2 **cans octopus**
- 1 **box of whole wheat table crackers**
     Chile pepper–and-garlic hot sauce, such as sriracha (optional)

MAKE IT: Cut the kale into 1-inch-wide strips, blanch in hot water, then cool in an ice bath. Set aside on a plate to dry. Drain the anchovies and place in a small bowl. Add the olive oil, lemon juice, and garlic. Use the back of a fork or a wooden spoon to mash together the dressing and add salt and pepper to taste. Dress the kale with the anchovy mixture in a mixing bowl. Drain the octopus. Set the crackers on a serving tray and top each with kale. Place 1 to 2 pieces of octopus on the kale and top with hot sauce, if desired. Serve immediately.

(Serves 4)

Ginger-Beet Soup

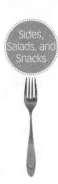

Beets might have a sugary reputation, but that's from their days as a popular canned food staple when sweetener was added to them. Believe it or not, but apples have 25 percent more sugar! This chilled soup is great any time of year, but it makes an especially refreshing meal or first course in the summer months. Beets are a great source of folate and betaine, both of which help reduce stress. Betaine, like folate, acts as a methyl donor, helping with the reactions that maintain our levels of SAM-e, a natural antidepressant made in our brains. Yogurt adds bone-building calcium and belly fat-fighting CLA and provides the needed fat for the absorption of fat-soluble vitamins. Beets get their red color from a molecule called betanin, which is a powerful antioxidant that protects the linings of our arteries from free radicals.

2 **bunches of beets, greens attached**
2 **tablespoons butter**
4 **cloves garlic, minced**
$^1/_4$ **cup minced fresh ginger**
1 **yellow onion, chopped**
4 **celery stalks, chopped**
1 **tomato, diced**
4 **carrots, chopped**
1 **cup red wine**
2 **cups water**
1 **lemon or lime, juiced**
 Salt and freshly ground black pepper
2 **cups whole-milk yogurt**

MAKE IT: Rinse the beets and set them in a large soup pot with water and boil for 45 minutes. Drain in a colander. Rinse with cool water and peel the skin by gently rubbing the beets; the peels will fall off with minimal effort. Place the butter in a soup pot and turn

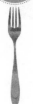

the heat on medium. Add the garlic and ginger and cook for 3 or 4 minutes, making sure not to burn the garlic. Add the onion and continue to cook until translucent. Add the celery and cook for another 3 minutes. Add additional butter to the pot, if necessary, to prevent the vegetables from burning. Add the beets, tomato, carrots, wine, water, and citrus juice. Cover and cook over medium heat for 35 minutes. Puree in batches in a blender, adding salt and pepper to taste. Serve the soup hot or cold, topped with a dollop of yogurt.

(Serves 4)

TOP 100 REASONS TO AVOID PROCESSED FOODS

Dioxin, one of the most toxic compounds known to man, routinely shows up in the meat of factory-farm animals due to poor feed controls.

Braised Red Cabbage Salad

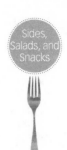

As you'll see with this recipe, cabbage is incredibly versatile. It's also an important staple of the Happiness Diet. By adding garlic and onion to the abundance of sulfur-containing molecules in red cabbage, you boost this dish's cancer-fighting powers.

3 tablespoons butter

2 cloves garlic, minced

1 small onion, chopped

1 head of red cabbage, chopped

1 cup red wine

2 tablespoons blackstrap molasses
    Salt and freshly ground black pepper

½ cup balsamic vinegar

2 green apples, chopped

1 cup crumbled goat cheese

MAKE IT: Place the butter in a saucepan over heat and, when melted, add the garlic and cook for 2 minutes, or until just browned. Add the onion and cook for about 5 minutes, until translucent. Add the cabbage, wine, and molasses and cover. Continue to cook over medium heat for about 15 minutes, or until the cabbage is soft. Remove the mixture from the heat and set aside in a bowl to cool. Add salt and pepper and vinegar to taste. Toss in the apples and goat cheese and serve.

(Serves 4)

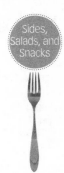

Butter Lettuce Salad

In this salad, butter lettuce (also known as Bibb or Boston lettuce) gets supercharged with the addition of radishes. Radishes belong to the Brassica family of vegetables, which includes nutrient superstars like broccoli and cabbage. Their peppery taste is due to a group of molecules called glucosinolates that block the formation of cancer cells.

1   **head butter lettuce**

5   **radishes**

2   **cloves garlic, minced**

White wine vinegar

Few tablespoons of olive oil

Salt and freshly ground black pepper

MAKE IT: Wash the lettuce, trim the ends, and set aside to dry. Slice the radishes thinly and set aside. Mix the garlic, vinegar, and olive oil together. Add salt and pepper to taste. Dress the salad in a large bowl, toss gently, and serve.

(Serves 2)

Belgian Endive Salad

Endive is a sleeper vegetable. Its slim, white appearance disguises the fact that it is jam-packed with nutrients and loaded with heart-healthy fiber. The addition of blue cheese and bacon give this salad a rich, hearty flavor and texture—you won't feel like you're eating "just a salad" but a full, satisfying meal.

- 2 cloves garlic, minced
- 1 lemon, juiced
- 1 tablespoon Dijon mustard
- 4 tablespoons olive oil
- Salt and freshly ground black pepper
- 1 handful of walnuts
- 5 heads endive
- 2 strips cooked bacon, cubed
- 3 ounces Stilton or other blue cheese, crumbled
- 1 Granny Smith apple, finely chopped

MAKE IT: To make the dressing, whisk together the garlic, lemon juice, mustard, and 3 tablespoons of the olive oil in a small glass bowl. Add salt and pepper to taste and set aside. Heat the remaining tablespoon of olive oil in a skillet on medium heat and add the walnuts; toast the nuts carefully, as they burn easily, over low heat for 3 to 5 minutes. When toasted and fragrant, remove the nuts from the pan and set aside. Trim the ends and any discolored leaves from the endive. Roughly chop the endive and place in a large bowl. Add the bacon, cheese, apple, and walnuts. Toss with dressing and serve immediately.

(Serves 4)

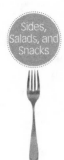
Raw Brussels Sprouts Salad

You may think this vegetable is way too powerful to eat raw, but you'll be surprised by just how well this simple salad stands up next to your favorite subtle fish or chicken recipes. Brussels sprouts boast more phytonutrient power than most other vegetables. Packed with folate, vitamin K, fiber, B$_6$, vitamin C, omega-3s, and tryptophan, they can be thought of as a multivitamin for your brain.

15   brussels sprouts

1   lemon, juiced

3   tablespoons olive oil

2   cloves garlic, minced

    Freshly ground black pepper

    Parmesan

MAKE IT: Chop the brussels sprouts into small pieces. Mix the lemon juice, olive oil, garlic, and pepper in a bowl to taste. Dress the brussels sprouts and then top with ample amounts of freshly grated Parmesan.

(Serves 4)

TOP 100 REASONS TO AVOID PROCESSED FOODS

University of Toronto researchers have found that perfluoroalkyls, chemicals that line food wrappers and repel grease, are entering the food supply. As these are associated with infertility, cancer, and elevated levels of bad cholesterol, this is not good news.

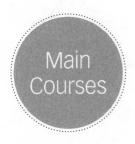

Roasted Chicken and Vegetables

There's nothing like the mouthwatering smell that fills the house when roasting a bird. And it's easy dish to prepare. This dish also makes excellent leftovers, which can be savored a day or two later with our Chicken Salad Sandwich. Good-bye, deli meat. Hello, hand-carved cuts. Chicken is a great source of complete protein, and it's particularly rich in tryptophan, which can boost mood. It is also packed with niacin that can decrease your risk of cognitive decline. Carrots provide lots of beta-carotene, and turnips are loaded with lutein, a top fat-soluble antioxidant that protects your vision.

1	medium (3–4 pounds) organic chicken
4	carrots
2	onions
1	turnip
$\frac{1}{2}$	cup olive oil
	Salt and freshly ground black pepper
2	lemons
2	sprigs fresh rosemary, chopped
$\frac{1}{4}$	bottle white wine or 2 cups chicken stock
$\frac{1}{2}$	stick butter

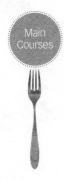

MAKE IT: Take the bird out of the refrigerator. Wash in cold water and pat dry. Let warm to room temperature for 30 minutes while you do rest of the prep. Preheat the oven to 400 degrees. Chop the carrots, onions, and turnip and place in a large bowl. Mix with the olive oil, salt and pepper to taste, and the juice from the lemons. Stuff the chicken with the rosemary, vegetables, and lemon rinds and place in a baking dish. Scatter the remaining veggies around the bird. Pour the wine or water over the bird. Smear a thick coat of butter on the bird. Place the pan on the middle rack of the oven and cook for at least 1 hour, or until juices run clear when you poke a hole in the chicken with a skewer or fork.

(Serves 2, with leftovers for chicken salad sandwiches)

Mexican Squid

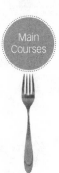

We're guessing squid probably hasn't been a regular rotation in your home, but we hope that will change with this quick and simple squid salad. It makes a perfect meal. Squid is loaded with copper, a rather rare trace nutrient, and taurine, an amino acid that is a calming, soothing neurotransmitter. It is also loaded with B_{12}. Avocados are packed with a great mix of fats and actually boost the absorption of carotenoids like beta-carotene and lycopene in the tomatoes by up to 400 percent.

1   avocado

4   tomatoes

½   red onion

1   red chile pepper (wear plastic gloves when handling)

2   tablespoons olive oil

1   lemon, juiced

    Salt and freshly ground black pepper

1   pound squid

2   tablespoons butter

MAKE IT: To make a salsa, chop the avocado into small cubes. Dice the tomatoes, onion, and chile pepper. Gently stir the vegetables together with the olive oil, lemon juice, and salt and pepper to taste. Meanwhile, cut the squid into thin strips. Melt the butter in a skillet and cook the squid for a few minutes on each side. Remove from the heat and set on top of the salsa. Add salt and pepper to taste. You may want to reserve a little lemon juice to squeeze over the final product.

(Serves 2)

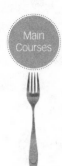

Slow Pork

Using low heat and longer cooking times yields pork that is tender and moist. Leftovers are great for tacos or salads. Use a slow cooker to nail this dish every time. It needs only a few minutes of prep and then can cook while you're at work, and when you return you'll have a meal ready to be devoured. Pork is a great source of thiamine, which the brain needs in order to keep its powerhouses running smoothly.

Salt and freshly ground black pepper
3 pound pork butt
6 medium apples, peeled and cubed
3 yellow onions, peeled and cubed
2½ cups chicken stock
Flour
1 cup chicken broth

MAKE IT: Salt and pepper the pork butt. Set it in a slow cooker and cover with the apples, onions, and stock. Turn the cooker on low and be prepared to be dazzled when you get home and find pork that literally falls apart it's so tender. To make gravy, put 1 cup of liquid from the slow cooker into a saucepan on medium-low heat. Sprinkle in a few pinches of flour. Using a whisk, stir the flour into the drippings. Keep adding flour and stirring until the gravy starts boiling and thickens. Serve over the pork.

(Serves 4)

Tuna Over Greens

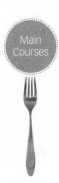

This is a delicious salad version of the classic tuna salad sandwich, and it works just as well for dinner as it does for lunch. It's simple and inexpensive. We recommend it with lemon vinaigrette, but truthfully you can eat it with nearly any of the dressings on page 218. You'll be getting a meal full of omega-3s and all the phytonutrients that leaves offer, promoting brain processing speed and fighting cancer and heart disease.

1 **lemon**

1 **can tuna**

½ **bag of mixed greens**

   Small handful of olive tapenade

   Small handful of capers

1 **fennel, thinly sliced**

   Lemon vinaigrette (see page 218)

   Salt and freshly ground black pepper

MAKE IT: Preheat the oven to 300 degrees. Thinly slice the lemon and place on a cookie sheet. Set in the oven and roast for 30 minutes. Scoop out the tuna and spread out over the mixed greens. Add the olive tapenade, capers, and fennel. Top with the lemon vinaigrette and add salt and pepper to taste.

(Serves TK)

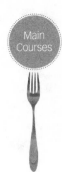

The HD Burger

Can the all-American burger, demonized as the centerpiece of cheap fast food, be good for you? Sure, just make 'em the HD way. First, we start with grass-fed beef, which eliminates the antibiotics, growth hormones, and general misery associated with beef from factory farms. You also get a naturally leaner beef high in healthy fats like the oft-touted omega-3s. The cheese is also full of healthy fats that will keep you satiated and prevent post-meal snacking. The whole grain bun is loaded with fiber and B-vitamins.

1¼   pounds grass-fed beef

     Salt and freshly ground black pepper

     Ketchup

     Mayonnaise

     Mustard

1   tomato

1   red onion

1   block of Vermont cheddar (blue cheese or gruyère will work, too)

1   head Boston lettuce

4   whole grain buns

MAKE IT: Pat the meat into four equal-size patties. Salt and pepper the beef and refrigerate for a minimum of an hour to let the burgers mold. Combine ketchup, mayonnaise, and mustard to taste to make your burger sauce, which should be creamy and slightly spicy. Refrigerate and prep the tomato, onion, and cheese by slicing these ingredients up. Remove the burgers from the fridge and grill for about 10 ten minutes. Toast buns on grill and top burgers with cheese until it melts. Remove burgers from grill. Top with the tomato and onion slices and lettuce. Slather the sauce on the top bun and enjoy.

(Serves 4)

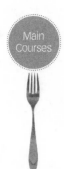
Grass-Fed Meatballs Marinara

Less is more when it comes to adding ingredients to this simple sauce and meatballs. Do make sure, however, that you're using the proper salt and pepper for seasoning, as you should with all of these recipes. You should be using at the least a quality kosher salt, if not sea salt. The bigger and more intense the grains of salt, the less you'll need to season. If you want to experiment with these meatballs, try tweaking one or two spices at a time. Another twist is doing a 50/50 mix of ground pork with ground beef. You'll have a much juicer meatball.

1½   **pounds grass-fed ground beef**
     Salt and freshly ground black pepper
2   **tablespoons butter**
½   **cup extra virgin olive oil**
4   **cloves garlic, diced**
1   **Spanish onion, diced**
3   **tablespoons chopped fresh thyme, or 1 tablespoon dried thyme**
½   **medium carrot, grated**
2   **(28-ounce) cans peeled whole tomatoes (gently hand crushed, with juice reserved)**
1   **cup red wine or beer (the darker the ale, the better)**
     Small chunk of Parmesan for grating

MAKE IT: Roll the ground beef into medium-size meatballs. Season with salt and pepper and set aside for 1 hour at room temperature before cooking. This will ensure the meat cooks evenly. In a 3-quart saucepan, heat 1 tablespoon of the butter and ¼ cup of the olive oil over medium heat until the butter is melted. Add the garlic and cook for 2 or 3 minutes, until just brown. Be careful to not burn the garlic—because if you do, you'll have to start all over. Add the onion and cook for 5 minutes, or until translucent. Add the

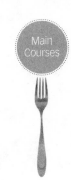

thyme and carrot and cook until the latter is soft (about 5 minutes). Add the tomatoes and their juice and bring the mixture to a boil, stirring often. Lower the heat and simmer the mixture for 30 minutes, or until it begins to thicken. In a skillet placed over medium heat, add the remaining olive oil and butter and cook until the butter melts. Add the wine or beer and meatballs and cover with a lid. Cook for about 10 minutes, until the meatballs are no longer pink inside. (Depending on the size of your skillet, you may need to cook the meatballs in batches.) Plate the meatballs and cover with the tomato sauce. Top with freshly grated Parmesan to taste.

(Serves 4)

TOP 100 REASONS TO AVOID PROCESSED FOODS

Buying processed foods is just another stop at the gas pump. The packaging, transport, fertilizer, and pesticides need to get processed food to your kitchen depends on billions and billions of barrels of oil.

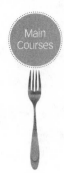

Steamed Mussels

This simple dish can be prepared in minutes. Mussels boast one of the highest concentrations of B_{12} in nearly any food. Ample B_{12} means the myelin insulation of your neurons will be protected and you'll stay sharp as you age. Mussels are also a great source of trace nutrients like zinc, iodine, and selenium—all of which are needed for a smooth-running brain. This preparation works great with clams, too.

12	mussels per person
2	cups white wine
1	cup water
2	tablespoons butter
2	cloves garlic
1	small onion, diced

MAKE IT: Thoroughly rinse the mussels in cold water to remove any sand. Then rinse once more for good measure, as a little sand often remains no matter how well you first rinsed. Discard cracked or opened mussels. Remove the "beards" with your fingers. Place the mussels in a large pot. Cover with the wine, water, butter, garlic, onion and your varietal flavoring of choice. The fluid should not completely cover the clams or mussels, but rather come up to about the halfway mark. Cover the pot and cook over high heat for 8 to 10 minutes, or until all mussels are open. Discard any closed shells, as they may not be cooked well enough inside to eat them safely. (Serves 12 mussels per person)

Make It Spicy:
2 jalapeño peppers or other favorite chile peppers, finely diced (wear plastic gloves when handling)

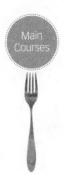

Make It Savory:
1 handful parsley, finely diced
2 links, cut coarsely, chorizo sausage

Make It Aromatic and Spicy:
2 tablespoons tarragon
3 Thai chile peppers, finely diced

Ginger Mackerel

Mackerel tops pretty much all other fish when it comes to omega-3s. But there is a blessing and a curse to this fish: Many avoid it because its rich oils can create a "fishy" taste. So, in walks ginger. Not only does the ginger tame any off notes, you also get the benefits of this spicy herb. Ginger is loaded with a set of powerful anti-inflammatory compounds called gingerols that protect the brain from free radicals, prevent the plaques that cause Alzheimer's disease, and reduce arthritic pain.

> Olive oil
> 2 pounds mackerel fillets
> 1 medium fresh ginger, grated
> 4 cloves garlic, minced
> 1/2 lemon, juiced
> 1/2 teaspoon kosher salt

MAKE IT: Coat the bottom of a glass ovenproof baking dish with olive oil. Rinse the fish fillets in water, then gently pat dry with paper towels. Place in the dish. Mix together the ginger, garlic, lemon juice, and salt. Cover the fillets with the mixture and let them sit for 10 minutes. Place under a broiler for 10 to 15 minutes, until the fish flakes.

(Serves 4)

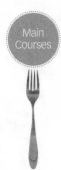

Main
Courses

Oven-Roasted Cod

Many people get intimidated by the thought of cooking fish. But oven roasting is a simple way to get it right every time. Cod is a wonderful source of complete protein and is especially high in tryptophan. Studies of this amino acid, the basic ingredient for making serotonin, show that it can help some people ditch the blues or with PMS. Instead of a supplement, cod is nature's top food source. You also get plenty of essential vitamins B_{12} and B_6, plus lots of EPA and DHA omega-3s, which are vital to heart and brain health. Cod is also full of selenium, which is needed for proper thyroid function and to make one of our most powerful intrinsic antioxidants, glutathione.

3	pats butter
4	medium fillets cod
1	cup white wine
2	tablespoons olive oil
3	cloves garlic, finely diced
$\frac{1}{2}$	teaspoon salt
	Freshly ground black pepper (optional)
3	sprigs tarragon

MAKE IT: Preheat the oven to 300 degrees. Smear 1 pat of butter in the bottom of an ovenproof baking dish. Place the fillets in the dish, skin side down. Pour the wine over the fish. Drizzle with olive oil, sprinkle on the garlic, then add the salt and pepper, if using. Place the tarragon on top of the fish. Cook covered in the oven for 18 to 22 minutes, until flaky.

(Serves 4)

Flawless Grilled Chicken

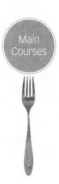

There is a really easy way of making chicken taste awesome all of the time. A simple process called brining (soaking the bird in a salt bath) creates a barrier that locks in moisture on the grill or in the oven. Among its many benefits, chicken is high in tryptophan, the amino acid that your body turns into the neurotransmitter melatonin, which promotes good sleep.

1   cup kosher salt, plus $\frac{1}{2}$ teaspoon

3   gloves garlic, minced

8   free-range organic boneless chicken thighs with skin

1   dozen free-range organic chicken legs

$\frac{1}{2}$ teaspoon freshly ground black pepper

MAKE IT: Add 4 quarts of water to a soup pot and place over high heat. When it comes to a boil, add 1 cup salt and the garlic. Simmer until the salt is dissolved. Remove the brine from the heat and let cool. Place all chicken parts in the brine, cover, and refrigerate overnight. When ready to cook, remove the chicken from the brine and pat dry with a paper towel. Sprinkle with the $\frac{1}{2}$ teaspoon salt and the pepper. (Or try your favorite rub or experiment with spices in your pantry—the real trick here is the brine.) Grill for 20 to 25 minutes over medium-high heat. If the legs have a significant amount of meat attached to them, they may take another 10 minutes to cook. Set aside to cool for 5 minutes before slicing or serving.

(Serves 4, with leftovers for Chicken Salad Sandwiches)

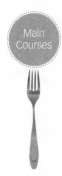

Chicken Salad Sandwiches

Remember that the best chicken salad sandwich is prepared intuitively; depending on which fresh leftovers you have on hand. If you have any vegetables left from the night before like Ginger Green Beans (page 183) or Brussels Spouts with Bacon (page 185), scoop a cup into the sandwich. If not, don't worry; your chicken salad will be delicious all the same. And remember to be careful not to overdo it with the mayo. You can always add more if needed, but you can't subtract mayo after you've overdone it.

Leftover chicken (see Roasted Chicken and Vegetables, page 195, or Flawless Grilled Chicken, above)

Mayonnaise

Dijon mustard

2 scallions, coarsely chopped (green parts only)

Small handful of whole pine nuts

Salt and freshly ground black pepper

8 pieces 100 percent whole wheat bread

1 head butter lettuce

1 fresh tomato, sliced

8 slices whole wheat bread, toasted

MAKE IT: Remove the chicken meat and skin from the bones and cut up. Set aside in a bowl. Add a few dollops of mayonnaise, depending on how much chicken you have, being careful not to make the chicken salad overly creamy. Add the mustard to taste. Stir in the scallions and pine nuts. Add salt and pepper to taste. Spread the chicken salad on a slice of bread and top with butter lettuce and tomato. Top with another slice of bread. Repeat until you have 4 sandwiches. Cut each in half to serve.

(Serves 4)

Perfect Pork Chops

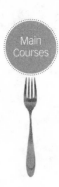

Pork chops can get pretty dried out. This recipe fixes that age-old problem. It's also a great main course for a family-style dinner. Just slice the pork after it's done cooking, place in a serving dish, and then top with the savory mustard sauce. These pork chops make wonderful leftovers and serve as a nice addition to a breakfast or atop a salad for lunch. Perfect Pork Chops also depend on getting the right pork. Pasture-raised pork will contain a healthier mix of fats and vitamin D. Pork also contains high concentrations of thiamine, which is used by all cells to make energy and is particularly important to the brain, and B_6, which helps make several key neurotransmitters.

4   **pork chops**
    Salt and freshly ground black pepper
3   **tablespoons olive oil**
2   **shallots, diced**
2   **tablespoons butter**
2   **cups white cooking wine**
3   **tablespoons Dijon mustard**
1   **tablespoon blackstrap molasses, maple syrup, or honey**

MAKE IT: Season both sides of the pork chops with salt and pepper to taste and drizzle with the olive oil. Set the chops on the counter for 1 hour before preparing the dish to bring them to room temperature. In a large skillet over medium heat, cook the shallots in butter until translucent. Add the wine, mustard, and molasses, syrup, or honey to the shallots and stir. Cook for 3 minutes, then add the pork chops and cover. Simmer for 25 minutes and remove from heat. To serve, let the pork chops rest for 5 minutes and then slice thinly and spoon the sauce over the top.

(Serves 4)

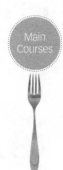
Happy Fish Salad Sandwiches

Like most recipes in this book, this salad can be altered endlessly and tweaked to your liking. Have a cup of kale left over from dinner? Dice it and mix into your fish salad for an added boost of flavor, fiber, and vitamin K. Or try adding some of your favorite hot sauce to this recipe and serve it on whole grain crackers as a snack or hors d'oeuvre. The options are endless.

1   (2-ounce) can anchovies
3   cloves garlic, diced
1   lemon, juiced
3   tablespoons olive oil
2   cans light chunk albacore tuna packed in olive oil
4   scallions, diced
    Salt and freshly ground black pepper
2   tablespoons mayonnaise
    White wine vinegar, to taste
8   slices whole wheat bread, toasted

MAKE IT: Remove the anchovies from the can and soak in a small bowl of water for 10 minutes—this will remove much of the salty fish flavor. Drain the water and add the garlic, lemon juice, and olive oil to the bowl. Muddle the mixture together with a fork until no large chunks of garlic or anchovies remain. Add the tuna, scallions, and salt and pepper to taste. Add the mayonnaise and the vinegar to taste. If the anchovy flavor is too strong, add more lemon juice and black pepper to dial it back. Spoon the salad on top of one slice of toasted bread and cover with a second slice. Repeat until you have 4 sandwiches. Cut each in half to serve.

(Serves 4)

The Happiness Diet EBLT

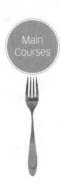

Adding an egg to the classic BLT sandwich boosts the content of choline, a nutrient we need for the production of new neurotransmitters. Some might scoff that this egg and bacon sandwich is high in saturated fat and cholesterol, but you now know that these are not the dietary demons they've been made out to be. They will, however, satiate you and prevent you from overeating throughout the day.

- 1 **tablespoon butter**
- 2 **pieces applewood-smoked bacon**
- 1 **free-range egg**
- 2 **slices whole wheat bread**
- 2 **tablespoons mayonnaise**
  Buttercup lettuce
- 1 **ripe heirloom tomato, sliced**
  Salt and freshly ground black pepper

MAKE IT: In a skillet, melt the butter and cook the bacon until it starts to get crispy; drain on paper towels and set aside. Fry the egg in the same pan (slightly runny is recommended). Toast the bread under the broiler on one side only. Spread a tablespoon of mayo on the toasted side of each slice of bread. Lay down a few slices of lettuce on one slice of the bread. Cover with the tomato slices, bacon, and egg. Season with salt and pepper to taste and top with the second slice of bread.

(Serves 1)

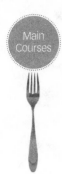

Happy Wild Salmon

Wild salmon is our top mood food for good reason. A few ounces contain more of the long-chained omega-3s DHA and EPA than does a handful of fish-oil pills. You also get an ample dose of B_6, B_{12}, zinc, copper, and selenium. Wild salmon is the top food source of vitamin D needed to beat the winter blues, fight cancer, and build strong bones. This delicious dill-yogurt sauce will make fish-eaters out of anyone (even your kids).

> **Salt and freshly ground black pepper**
> 2 **pounds wild-caught salmon steaks, deboned**
> 1 **cup whole-milk plain yogurt**
> **Generous pinch of brown sugar**
> 1 **lemon, juiced**
> 1 **tablespoon Dijon mustard**
> 1 **tablespoon olive oil**
> **A few sprigs dill (optional)**

MAKE IT: Sprinkle salt and pepper over salmon steaks and let sit for a minimum of 30 minutes at room temperature. Preheat the oven to 375 degrees. In a small bowl, mix together the yogurt, brown sugar, lemon juice, mustard, olive oil, additional salt (if desired), and dill, if using. Bake the salmon for 10 to 15 minutes in a baking pan. Remove the salmon and let sit for 10 minutes. Top salmon steaks with half of the sauce, and pour the remainder of the sauce into a serving vessel.

(Serves 4)

Grass-Fed Balsamic Flank Steak

People wonder whether the extra few dollars spent on naturally raised, grass-fed beef is worth it. That conventionally raised steak might look similar, but it's it not. Grass-fed meat is lower in total fat but much higher in health-promoting omega-3 fats and belly-fat-blasting CLA. Eating grass-fed beef, following the HD rules, is a delicious way to protect your brain health.

- 1 **pound flank steak**
  Salt and freshly ground black pepper, to taste
- 1 **tablespoon olive oil**
- 2 **tablespoons butter**
- 1 **small shallot, minced**
- ½ **cup balsamic vinegar**
- 2 **tablespoons blackstrap molasses**

MAKE IT: Coat the flank steaks on both sides with salt and pepper. Drizzle with the olive oil and let sit for 45 minutes at room temperature. In a saucepan, melt the butter and add the shallot; cook until fragrant. Then add the vinegar and molasses. Simmer for 3 minutes and set aside. In a dry skillet, cook the steak on medium-high for 5 minutes on each side. Remove from the heat and let sit 5 to 10 minutes. Slice thinly against the grain. Place the steak slices in a small bowl and toss with the sauce.

(Serves 4)

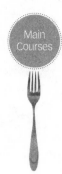
Spicy Fish Stew

Here's a simple, refreshing recipe that works well with the vast options of white fish—cod, sea bass, fluke—sold by many fishmongers or markets. You can also substitute scallops or shellfish, like clams or mussels, if you like. While you're enjoying the rich broth, smile because you are getting minerals like iodine, selenium, and zinc that are fundamental to good moods and clear thinking.

2	bundles asparagus
$3/4$	pound broccoli
4	tablespoons olive oil
1	tablespoon butter
4	cloves garlic, minced
2	large leeks, chopped
2	tablespoons sriracha sauce (Asian hot sauce)
2	tablespoons sesame oil
3	cups white cooking wine
2	lemons, juiced
$1\frac{1}{2}$	pounds of your favorite white fish, cut into $1\frac{1}{2}$-inch cubes
	Salt and freshly ground black pepper

MAKE IT: Snap the asparagus into 1½-inch-long spears. Set aside. Separate the florets from the broccoli stalk. Set aside. In a saucepan over medium-high heat, add the olive oil and butter and heat until the butter melts. Reduce the heat to medium and add the garlic. Cook for about a minute, or until the garlic becomes fragrant. And the leeks and cook for about 5 minutes, or until they soften and become transparent. Add the asparagus, broccoli, sriracha sauce, sesame oil, wine, and lemon juice. Cover and cook for 5 to 8 minutes, until the broccoli and asparagus begin to turn bright green and soften. While cooking, taste the broth and season with sriracha to your desired level of spiciness. Add the fish and cook about 6 minutes, until flaky. Remove from the heat and serve.

(Serves 2)

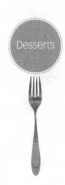

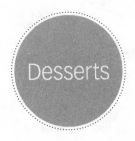

Lemon Macaroons

Coconut fat got a bad rap, but that reputation is undeserved. Coconut's medium-chain fats enhance your body's fat-burning capacity and production of ketones, the only other fuel your brain can burn beside glucose. Lemon zest powers these with liminoids aplenty, plus citrus flavonoids that protect the brain.

- 3 **eggs**
- 3 **cups shredded coconut**
- 2 **tablespoons lemon zest**

MAKE IT: Preheat the oven to 375 degrees. Vigorously whisk the eggs in a large bowl. Using your hands, mix in the shredded coconut and lemon zest. Mold about a tablespoon of the mixture into small balls and place on a butter-greased baking sheet. Bake for 18 to 22 minutes, or until golden on top.

(Makes about 30 cookies, serves 15)

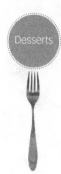

Sweet Sundae

This ice cream sundae does contain ample amounts of sugar. But if you are like us, you're likely not giving up ice cream, so we use it to transport the phytonutrients from berries plus omega-3s, toco-trienols, and tocopherols (vitamin E) from walnuts and almonds, all of which protect your brain. Even better if you can find a grass-fed ice cream. The CLA in grass-fed dairy makes this an ice cream sundae that could reduce belly fat.

1	**pint vanilla ice cream**
1	**cup berries**
$^1/_2$	**cup walnuts**
$^1/_2$	**cup slivered almonds**

MAKE IT: Place all the ingredients in a bowl. Mash together. Sit down on the couch and enjoy a bowl in silent bliss with a few friends.

(Serves 4)

TOP 100 REASONS TO AVOID PROCESSED FOODS

When the world's largest food processor discovered how popular diets focusing on natural meats and low carbohydrates have become, they developed a program to create products . . . for a movement that is all about not eating processed foods.

Happy Watermelon

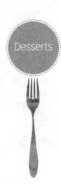

It's difficult to find a sweeter summertime treat than a perfectly ripe watermelon, nature's tastiest alternative to the sugary treats that line our convenience stores and supermarkets. You will be amazed by how citrus juice unlocks the sweet watermelon taste, even if your melon is slightly underripe. This refreshing dish makes a perfect side salad or dessert on a hot summer night.

1	watermelon
4–6	limes, or 3–5 lemons, or your own combination of the two

MAKE IT: Cut the watermelon into cubes and place in a large bowl. Toss with the lime or lemon juice or a combination of the fruits. After a few tries, you'll figure out which taste is right for you. If you like the dish chilled, refrigerate for at least an hour and serve.

(Serves 10)

Dressings: How to Win Best Dressed

Knowing how to make vegetables consistently taste good is as simple as understanding how to make a delicious vinaigrette. The basic formula is two or three parts oil to one part acid. You might think of it as simply "salad dressing," but chefs have been making this simple concoction long before bottled mixtures appeared on grocery store shelves. Vinaigrettes literally take just minutes to whip up and cost pennies on the dollar compared to their store-bought counterparts. Not surprisingly, the mass-produced stuff is typically full of inflammatory omega-6 fatty acids, high fructose corn syrup, and preservatives. Here are a few simple vinaigrette recipes that you can whip up in a flash and that will expose your vegetables to the fats you need to absorb their nutrients.

Lemon juice + olive oil + salt + black pepper = lemon vinaigrette

This bright and tangy dressing is delicious on raw vegetables like carrots and broccoli. It's also excellent on steamed vegetables such as asparagus or on a bitter green like arugula, topped with Parmesan. Use the juice of 1 lemon and season the rest according to taste.

Chopped fresh tarragon + olive oil + sherry vinegar + minced shallot + salt + black pepper = tarragon vinaigrette

This fresh, light dressing will add an herbaceous kick to raw vegetables like cucumbers, tomatoes, carrots, and mixed greens. Use 1–2 sprigs of tarragon and 1 shallot and season the rest according to taste.

Chopped anchovy fillets + olive oil + lemon juice + minced garlic + salt + black pepper = anchovy vinaigrette

This savory vinaigrette pairs well with crisp raw vegetables like green beans, lettuce, or shaved asparagus or roasted vegetables like potatoes and kale. Use 1 can anchovies, the juice of 1 lemon, a few cloves of garlic, and the rest to taste.

Fresh minced ginger + olive oil + sherry vinegar + fresh lime juice + salt + black pepper = ginger vinaigrette

This spicy, tangy topping is perfect on sautéed mushrooms and bitter greens (like bok choy and mustard greens) as well as Asian-style salads. Use a small piece of fresh ginger, 1–1½ limes, and the rest to taste.

Grainy mustard + apple cider or sherry vinegar + olive oil + minced shallots + salt + vinegar = Dijon vinaigrette

This tart and savory dressing is delicious on simple salads (like butter lettuce and radishes) and pretty much anything else. Try it on roasted beets. Use 1 tablespoon of mustard, 2 shallots, and the rest to taste.

Fresh chopped basil + minced garlic + olive oil + white wine or champagne vinegar + salt + black pepper = basil vinaigrette

This fresh and sweet vinaigrette pairs beautifully with fresh tomatoes as well as grilled or roasted vegetables like parsnips and summer squash. Use 3–4 sprigs of basil, 2 garlic cloves, and the rest to taste.

Fish sauce + rice wine vinegar + lime juice + minced garlic + minced chile peppers + water + sugar to taste = Asian vinaigrette

This vinaigrette starts out with a staple Vietnamese condiment as its base—fermented fish sauce—and lends a pungent, spicy-sweet kick to heartier roasted vegetables like cauliflower and brussels sprouts. Use ½ cup fish sauce, 1 lime, 2–3 cloves garlic, a few small red peppers, and the rest to taste.

Red wine vinegar + olive oil + shallots + Dijon mustard + salt + black pepper = red wine vinaigrette

This slightly sour vinaigrette is incredibly versatile—try it on sweet roasted vegetables like golden beets or on bitter sautéed greens.

Fresh tomatoes + diced shallots + minced garlic + olive oil + sherry vinegar + salt + black pepper = tomato vinaigrette

This fresh, juicy dressing can be tossed with salad greens or makes a great topping on grilled veggies like zucchini and summer squash. Use 2 really ripe tomatoes (diced), 1 shallots, 1 clove garlic, and the rest to taste.

Diced cooked bacon + olive oil + apple cider vinegar + Dijon mustard + salt + black pepper = bacon vinaigrette

A rich, savory topping that's great on bitter sautéed greens like kale, collard greens, or spinach. Use 4 pieces bacon, 1 tablespoon mustard, and the rest to taste.

TOP 100 REASONS TO AVOID PROCESSED FOODS

New research shows that the MAD life is so depleted of nutrients that today's babies may come out of the womb with a thrifty gene turned on that makes them more likely to gain weight. That's because from their bodies' viewpoint, the world outside of the womb is devoid of the nutrients their brains and bodies need. So they come into the world predisposed to make the most of any food they can get their hands on.

Epilogue

Spreading Happiness

At the end of your fork is a decision that is greater than simply your own happiness. You hold a power at every meal to help spread a smile across America. Just as a ripple spreads out across a pond when you jump in it on a hot summer day—you can spread happiness.

If we all made some simple choices at mealtimes; if we paused and took some time to appreciate our food, the land that it was cultivated from, and the people who grew it—things would change. And things are changing. A wave is cresting in America; we are becoming increasingly aware of our food. The number of farmers' markets is growing exponentially. There is even a giant rooftop farm in Brooklyn. The power behind these swift changes is our food choices.

Good food, healthy food for America is something that people of all political and economic stripes should agree on. We should all desire to give our children food that grows brains ready to engage with the world and poised to learn all that our schools have to offer. So next time you pick up your fork, remember that you're not just making a decision that impacts your mood and waistline—you're also choosing what kind of country you want to live in.

Bonus

Top 100 Reasons to Avoid Supplements

Walk into your neighborhood drugstore,

and you'll find an entire section devoted to supplements. The labels on the bottles promise they'll boost brain power, improve mood, fight cancer, help you sleep, and even make your skin, nails, and hair look younger.

As time-crunched and stressed out as we all are, quick fixes can be appealing. But it's important to understand that vitamins in supplement form are dramatically different from those found in food—and your body knows the difference. Take vitamin E, for example: As we stated earlier, if you eat a variety of leafy greens and whole grains, you'll get eight different forms of this nutrient. Yet most supplements and fortified foods contain only one synthetic form of vitamin E known as alpha-tocopherol, which research shows actually *increases* the risk of cancer and heart disease.

And because the supplement industry is unregulated by the FDA, claims of safety and efficacy aren't approved or endorsed by any government agency. The FDA has the power to stop sales only after a product is deemed unsafe—by trial and error on consumers. Over nineteen thousand people got seriously ill (more than a hundred died) before the FDA was able to ban the herbal weight-loss stimulant ephedra.

Many health experts suggest taking a multivitamin as an "insurance policy" to make up for dietary deficiencies, yet studies have failed to prove conclusively that multivitamins will make you healthier. In an attempt to give pills and powders some credibility, the National Center for Complementary and Alternative Medicine (part of the National Institutes of Health) has spent about one billion dollars on research—and yet, with the exception of fish oil and vitamin D, no supplement has been scientifically proven to improve health.

Here are one hundred more reasons to get your nutritional needs met through food, not pills:

1. Snake-oil salesman really did exist. In the 1800s, concoctions like Tex Bailey's Rattle Snake Oil and Rattlesnake Bill's Liniment and Monster Brand Snake Oil were promoted to treat everything from muscle spasms to frostbite to cancer. Chemical analysis later proved that these "medicines" were little more than crude mixtures of mineral oil and additives like turpentine.

2. Utah Senator Orin Hatch, who reports taking daily vitamins, receives campaign contributions from manufacturers like Herbalife, Metabolife, Rexall Sundown Naturals, and Nu Skin Worldwide. He lobbied for legislation that limits the FDA's regulatory power over supplements. Utah is the only state with a supplement trade association; supplements are its third-largest industry.

3. A study published in the *Archives of Internal Medicine* followed more than 160,000 postmenopausal women and found that multivitamin use had "little or no influence" on cancer or longevity, leading the authors to recommend, "Nutritional efforts should remain the principle focus of chronic disease prevention."

4. Smokers who obtain their vitamin E from supplements have an increased risk of lung cancer, while those who get their vitamin E from produce have a decreased risk.

5. Studies have linked multivitamin use by young children to an increased risk of developing asthma and food allergies.

6. No one is required to study the safety of supplements before they go to market.

7. While you've likely heard about Chinese raw ingredients being frequently contaminated with chemicals and toxins like melamine, you may not know that China manufactures 90 percent of the world's vitamin C supplements.

8. The herbal stimulant and weight-loss supplement ephedra was "officially" banned by the FDA in 2004, but it's unclear what that really means because you can still purchase it from Internet vendors. In other words, you can't even trust that a supplement you're buying hasn't already been banned.

9. In 2009, fourteen varieties of the weight-loss supplement Hydroxycut were recalled after twenty-three reports of severe adverse reactions like liver damage . . . and death. Hydroxycut was reformulated and is now back on the market.

10. Supplements come in much higher dosages than are found in food. You'd need to eat five whole cantaloupes to equal a standard 1,000-milligram vitamin C supplement.

11. According to multiple studies, saw palmetto, a popular herb used to treat enlarged prostates, works no better than a placebo.

12. Supplements such as garlic are often coated in plastic that contains phthalates, which have been linked to ADHD, allergies, weight gain, birth defects, and cancer.

13. Zicam Cold Remedy nasal gel and swabs were pulled off shelves in 2009 after reports that the products were linked to a permanent loss of smell.

14. Independent testing company ConsumerLab.com discovered that many vitamins labeled "natural" are actually synthetic.

15. People who take vitamin A supplements are at an increased risk of hip fracture.

16. When thiamine supplements are given to cancer patients, they can actually fuel tumor growth and interfere with chemotherapy.

17. It's estimated that the FDA has the capacity to examine only 1 percent of supplement shipments that arrive in US ports.

18. Colloidal silver is marketed as an infection fighter and immune booster. Overuse of it can also turn some people's skin permanently blue—giving new meaning to the term "feeling blue."

19. Of 324 brands of multivitamins recently tested by the FDA, 320 were contaminated with lead, a neurotoxin.

20. The herb ginkgo biloba is touted for its ability to boost brain function, but every study to date that has tested its efficacy has come up negative.

21. The herbal cold and flu product Airborne became an overnight success after the schoolteacher who created it went on Oprah. Two years later, the company admitted its sole clinical trial was faulty and as a result paid $23.3 million as part of a class action lawsuit.

22. "Proprietary blend" is a fancy way of saying you're not allowed to know how much of each ingredient is included in the bottle.

23. Vitamin A and beta-carotene supplements are linked to an increase in a smoker's risk of dying of cancer by 60 percent.

24. In 2008, the FDA reported that Total Body Formula liquid multivitamins contained two hundred times more selenium and seventeen times more chromium than indicated on the label. As a result, some people who took them suffered from hair loss, muscle cramps, diarrhea, joint pain, and fatigue.

25. Men who regularly take calcium supplements have a slightly greater risk of developing prostate cancer.

26. The FDA has tested only a fraction of the hundreds of the manufacturing facilities that produce America's supplements.

27. Folic acid supplements are linked to an increased risk of developing breast cancer in women. We're not suggesting you forgo folic acid supplementation while trying to get pregnant or during pregnancy, if that's what your physician advises, but that over the long haul taking folic acid is linked to breast cancer. It's a good reason to avoid processed foods that are supplemented with this vitamin.

28. The sleep aid L-tryptophan was pulled off the market after it was linked to a blood disorder called eosinophilia-myalgia syndrome that killed at least 37 people and permanently disabled more than 1,500 others.

29. Calcium, zinc, and magnesium supplements are known to block the absorption of iron, which is needed to build neurotransmitters like serotonin.

30. Each year, the American Association of Poison Control Centers files more than 126,000 reports of poisonings from supplements.

31. Valerian root, an herbal supplement used to treat insomnia, is often contaminated with cadmium and lead—heavy metals that accumulate in the body and cause brain damage.

32. Taking 500 milligrams of vitamin B_6 per day can lead to nerve damage in the arms and legs.

33. Soy isoflavones are promoted for improving menopausal hot flashes, lowering cholesterol, increasing bone density, and reducing the risk of breast cancer; however, these benefits have never been proven.

34. The International Olympic Committee tested 240 supplements and found that 20 percent of them were contaminated with banned substances like steroids.

35. Probiotic supplements can contain as little as 7 percent of the good bacteria advertised on the bottle.

36. Twenty percent of fish oil is manufactured in China—yet there's no way to know from where yours came from reading the label.

37. The label claim of "natural" is meaningless. It has no universal definition, and, when you think about it, that means everything is "natural." Everything, no matter how processed, still comes from "nature."

38. Unlike dietary magnesium, synthetic magnesium can cause diarrhea and abdominal cramping, according to the Institute of Medicine.

39. The children's vitamin L'il Critters Gummi Vites, sold at Costco and Walmart, was found to contain 2.5 micrograms of lead per serving.

40. A study published in the *New England Journal of Medicine* found that echinacea in no way helps to prevent or treat a cold.

41. A herbal supplement for prostate health called PC-SPES contained DES, an artificial estrogen banned in 1971, and some men who took the supplement suffered enlarged breasts, shrunken genitals, and deadly blood clots.

42. Liqiang 4, a dietary supplement marketed as a natural way to help control blood sugar, contains glyburide, a prescription medication for diabetes that can cause life-threateningly low blood sugar if not taken properly.

43. Bitter orange, often found in ephedra-free products, contains synephrine, a chemical cousin of ephedra, and causes the same side effects that increase the risk of heart attack, stroke, and death.

44. Metabolife, a top producer of ephedra supplements prior to the 2004 FDA ban, was founded by Michael Ellis, a former police officer, shortly after he served time for producing methamphetamines.

45. A large study on people with arthritic knees found that neither glucosamine, chondroitin, or a combination of the two, eased pain.

46. Supplements like vitamin C and E taken before a workout counter the benefits of exercise. That's because you actually want a fair amount of free radicals bouncing around when you exercise. That's what your body recovers from. When taken before a workout, these antioxidants prevent that from happening.

47. Despite many well-designed studies, there's no evidence that zinc lozenges help treat a cold. And using them for longer than six weeks can cause a copper deficiency, which can lead to anemia.

48. Acai berry supplements (advertised as having antiaging and metabolism-boosting properties) have been found to be contaminated with Viagra, which can cause heart attacks and stroke.

49. Prozac has been found in some weight-loss supplements.

50. Phenolphthalein has been found in weight-loss supplements. It can cause mutations in DNA. It has also been linked to cancer.

51. Rimonabant has been identified in some weight-loss supplements, which has been linked to depression and suicide.

52. The FDA lists seventy-one weight-loss supplement brands—like Slim Up, 2 Day Diet, and Super Fat Burner—to be wary of due to product adulteration.

53. Kava supplements, marketed to treat anxiety, insomnia and PMS, often include the leaves and stems of the plant, which contain the toxic alkaloid pipermethystine, known to cause severe liver damage.

54. The New York City Department of Health and Mental Hygiene found lead levels ten thousand times the FDA limit in the supplement Vita Breath.

55. Chinese star anise tea used to treat colic in infants has led to numerous reports of seizures and vomiting, likely due to the

addition of Japanese star anise, which contains the toxin sikimitoxin, which causes these symptoms and is lethal at higher doses.

56. Half of weight-loss formulations containing chromium tested by ConsumerLabs.com contained hexavalent chromium, a known carcinogen.

57. Aristolochic acid, found in many weight-loss pills, is a human carcinogen.

58. Most garlic supplements don't contain allicin, the compound in fresh garlic that fights bacteria and viral infection.

59. Since 1983, the number of adverse events related to herbal supplements reported to the American Association of Poison Control Centers have increased by more than 800 percent.

60. The supplement Seng Jong Tzu Tong Tan produced by Herbal Science International contains human placenta.

61. Despite what you may have heard, there's no evidence that vitamin C improves immunity.

62. Megadoses of vitamin B_3 (niacin) are prescribed by physicians to lower cholesterol, but its side effects include high blood sugar, liver damage, and interference with certain medications. Side effects from a proper diet and exercise are nonexistent.

63. The supplement Seasilver touted itself as a cure for 648 ailments, including cancer and heart disease, until the FDA and FTC fined the company $120 million. Now it's sold as SeaAloe.

64. NeuroBliss, a supplement beverage that claims to enhance mood and improve memory, contains sodium benzoate, a preservative that is neurotoxic. If that's not a mood killer, we don't know what is.

65. If you take supplements to avoid the pharmaceutical industry, you're out of luck. Pfizer, for example, owns the Centrum brands of vitamins.

66. Supplement beverages that claim to improve brain function, like Vitaminwater's Spark, are made with crystalline fructose, which is even more fattening than high fructose corn syrup.

67. Contrary to the popular belief that supplemental antioxidants provide health benefits, an analysis published in the *Journal of the American Medical Association* revealed that supplemental beta-carotene, vitamin A, and vitamin E increase the risk of death by up to 16 percent.

68. Dehydroepiandrosterone (DHEA), a popular supplement you can pick up in GNC, Vitamin Shoppe, or Walmart, is a potent steroid hormone that can cause hair loss in men and facial hair growth in women and that has been linked to breast and prostate cancer.

69. The FDA issued a warning in November 2009 regarding a sexual enhancement supplement called Stiff Nights. Marketed as an all-natural product, it illegally contained a potent drug sulfoaildenafil, which can cause dangerously low blood pressure.

70. Many supplement manufacturers are charlatans just like the original snake-oil salesmen. Herbalife International, for example, sells supplements in seventy-two countries and racked up $3.8 billion in sales in 2009. Founder Mark Hughes claimed he was inspired by his mother's death from an accidental prescription diet pill overdose. With ephedra's ban due to toxic side effects, Herbalife's ephedra-based diet products are now implicated in the deaths of hundreds of dieters, a story similar to the one spun by Hughes about his mother.

71. Body-building supplements like Advanced Muscle Science's Arom-X contain aromatase inhibitors that can decrease sperm count, cause kidney failure, and inhibit bone growth.

72. No major medical group or organization promotes taking a daily multivitamin.

73. FCC Products, Inc. distributed ginseng supplements contaminated with the pesticides procymidone and quintozene, which disrupt sexual development and promote the formation of tumors.

74. While the FDA is charged with policing (but not regulating) supplements, the agency has been involved in bribery scandals and charged with helping manufacturers falsify data.

75. Vitamin A produced in China and destined for addition to baby formula in Europe was found to be contaminated with *Enterobacter sakazakii*, a toxic bacteria that kills up to 80 percent of the infants it infects.

76. Sodium chlorite, the main active ingredient in Miracle Mineral Supplement, is converted to chlorine dioxide—a powerful industrial-strength bleach used for waste water treatment—when MMS is mixed with citric acid or juice as per instructions on the bottle.

77. The lack of regulation of herbal supplements means a teenager can order the powerful hallucinogen *Salvia divinorum* from the Internet.

78. Nature's Way Complete Multivitamin Alive! Men's Energy multivitamin is labeled as a "high potency, whole food energizer with 26 fruits and vegetables," but the majority of the nutrients are the same synthetic versions used in other multivitamins.

79. The recalled herbal insomnia remedy Sleeping Buddha contained the prescription sedative estazolam, which carries a risk of addiction, depression, and cognitive impairment.

80. Ginseng is regularly contaminated with lead because it is dried out in China by being driven over by trucks—the contamination comes from the tailpipe exhaust.

81. The FDA cannot force a manufacturer to remove tainted products from the marketplace.

82. After the discovery of widespread data fabrication by supplement manufacturers, the Therapeutic Goods Administration—the Australian equivalent of the FDA—had to recall more than 1,500 products.

83. Metabolife received fifteen thousand reports of adverse events that it did not report to the FDA.

84. Pissing your money away? That's pretty much what you are doing with most vitamins and supplements, because they are quickly filtered out by your kidneys. The dark yellow urine that comes after ingesting a multivitamin comes from B_2, also used as a food coloring.

85. Combining prescription medications for depression with "mood-boosting" supplements puts you at risk for dangerous drug interactions that can trigger mood changes, high blood pressure, headaches, heart arrhythmias, and liver failure.

86. U-Prosta, a "natural" supporter of prostrate health, was found to contain terazosin, a prescription medication used for treatment of an enlarged prostate that can cause fainting and low blood pressure.

87. Protein powder supplements have been contaminated with salmonella, an unfriendly bacteria that can cause bloody diarrhea and destroy heart valves.

88. Every year, roughly thirty-three thousand kids are sickened when they take their parents' iron supplements. A mere 200 milligrams of iron can be fatal to a child.

89. Believe you can trust supplement manufacturers? Although often more altruistic than the big pharmaceutical companies, they aren't always so. Take the story behind "the Greatest Vitamin in the World." This pill was formulated by Doug Grant, who was convicted in 2009 of killing his wife by drugging her with Ambien and drowning her in their bathtub. He teamed with infomercial pitchman and multilevel marketer Don Lapre,

who was warned by the FDA in 2005 and 2006 for making health claims, and investigated by the FTC, the Better Business Bureau, the US Postal Service Inspector General, and the IRS.

90. The Que She herbal supplement available on the Internet and at retail outlets like Sacred Journey in Lawrence, Kansas, contain three banned drugs—fenfluramine (of Fen-Phen fame), sibutramine, and ephedrine. To counteract the rapid heart rate, increased blood pressure, and anxiety from this cocktail, the manufacturers add propranolol, a prescription blood pressure medication that can cause depression and trigger asthma.

91. Prior to hitting shelves, a supplement must be assessed by the FDA only if it contains a "new dietary ingredient," defined as a dietary supplement not marketed in the United States prior to October 15, 1994. While it is left to manufacturers to determine if an ingredient warrants FDA notification, no comprehensive list of supplements (prior to this date) exists.

92. Saint-John's-wort has demonstrated efficacy in the treatment of some forms of depression and is regulated as a prescription medication in Germany. Laboratory tests of Saint-John's-wort supplements in the United States show contamination with cadmium and lead that can lead to mental impairment and lower concentration.

93. The combination of iron-fortified foods and iron in supplements has some researchers concerned about iron overload, leading to excess free radical production and an increased risk of colon cancer.

94. Birth defects can be caused by the mislabeling of supplements, like a swap of vitamin A for vitamin C that led to a recall in Canada. Vitamin A in concentrations as low as 10,000 IU, the amount in just two or three pills of many multivitamins, increases the risk by 2.5 times of having a baby with a cleft lip, a cleft palate, hydrocephalus, or a heart malformation.

95. A study of the male enhancement supplement Enzyte published in the *Archives of Internal Medicine* found that young, healthy men had changes in their heart rhythm (called a QTc increase) that is the harbinger of a fatal arrhythmia. Prescription medications that cause QTc increases get a "black box" warning from the FDA and require regular monitoring by a physician.

96. Supplements that boast memory-boosting power generally make this claim using single, small trials and include ingredients that don't even make it past the blood-brain barrier to get into the brain.

97. Spending money on supplements that have no evidence they promote happiness means less money to buy Happiness Diet foods, which have ample evidence they do.

98. Tocotrienols, the forms of vitamin E emerging as the most neuroprotective, aren't ingredients in the majority of vitamin E supplements.

99. Phosphatidylserine is a supplement marketed to improve brain function, though an FDA evaluation of human trials found no evidence of this claim. Early formulations were derived from cow brains—a practice that stopped due to concerns of mad cow disease.

100. Soladek is a supplement that claims to treat "hypo and avitaminosis, rickets, growth, dentition, lactation, fractures, infection . . . aging and pregnancy." It was found to contain toxic levels of vitamin A and 600,000 IU of vitamin D per vial—one thousand times the Recommended Dietary Allowance. The FDA issued a warning after reports of severe adverse events from its use.

Appendix

A Complete Guide to the Fats in Food

Fats serve our body in three ways: as energy sources, as building blocks of our cells, and as precursors for signals that regulate brain growth, inflammation, hunger, and blood sugar. Your brain is mainly fat and so is your endocrine system, the part of your body that produces hormones like insulin, cortisol, testosterone, and leptin that regulate mood, energy metabolism, and growth. The mix of fats in the diet are organized into chemical structures known as polyunsaturated, monounsaturated, and saturated. As you're about to see, they're much more complicated than "good and bad." They're nearly as complex as you are, and shunning fat from the diet is a terrible mistake.

Polyunsaturated

Omega-3s

ALA: Alpha-linolenic acid is the simplest omega-3 fat. ALA is found in the leaves of plants and is the major fat found in kale, brussels sprouts, and broccoli. It is especially concentrated in flaxseed, purslane, and walnuts. You'll also find ALA in eggs and meat from pasture-raised animals.

Plants use this special fatty acid to convert sunlight into energy and it is the most abundant fat on the planet. ALA is used to make the specialized omega-3 fatty acids important for brain and heart health, but humans are inefficient at this conversion. That's why meat (like fish and pasture-raised eggs and beef) is the best source of the most important omega-3s (see below).

SDA: Stearidonic acid is the intermediate step in the conversion of ALA to the longer chain omega-3s (see EPA and DHA below) that are essential to staving off brain disorders, heart disease, obesity and diabetes. You'll find SDA in seafood, especially mackerel, and spirulina (blue-green algae) as well as in blackcurrant, borage, and echium oils.

EPA: Eicosapentaenoic acid plays a critical role in cooling inflammation. EPA is used by your body to make potent anti-inflammatory compounds that keep blood vessels relaxed and prevent blood clots. The more EPA in your diet, the lower the concentration of pro-inflammatory omega-6 fats (see below) in your cells. Our bodies can make EPA from ALA, but not very efficiently, which is why you need it in your diet. Low EPA is linked to depression, suicide, diabetes, and heart disease. EPA is found in fatty fish like sardines, salmon, mackerel; shellfish like shrimp, oysters, clams; and grass-fed ruminants like beef, bison, sheep, and goats.

DPA: Docosapentaenoic acid is a long chain omega-3 fat that protects neurons. It is the intermediate step between EPA and DHA. More DPA in your blood lowers your risk of heart disease, but DPA's role in our body is largely unstudied. DPA is present in seal oil and most fatty fish like sardines, salmon, mackerel, and herring.

DHA: Docosahexaenoic acid is the most abundant omega-3 fat in your brain and makes 50 percent of the fat in neurons. Our brains use DHA to make potent hormones called neuroprotectins and resolvins that combat inflammation. DHA also blocks the signals that cause brain cells to die during stress. Studies suggest that you need to eat about two grams a day to get optimal concentrations in your tissues. Low levels of DHA are associated with depression, bipolar disorder, ADHD, and Alzheimer's disease. The most concentrated source of DHA is in cold-water fatty fish like salmon, mackerel, and sardines. Vegetarians can get DHA from certain algae.

Omega-6s

LA: The omega-6s are your body's alarm system. They trigger your body's inflammatory pathways which mobilize immune cells and lead to things like swelling, redness, and pain. These are healthy responses to injury or sickness that protect us. But too much linoleic acid (LA) in the diet promotes unnecessary inflammation leading to chronic illness. LA and the other omega-6 fats compete with omega-3 fats for regulatory enzymes. More LA causes more oxidative stress on the body and brain. LA is the main fat from corn, soy, cottonseed, safflower, and sunflower oil and today we get more calories from LA than ever before in history.

GLA: Gamma linoleic acid helps cool off inflammation. A lot of people castigate all omega-6s, but it's more complicated that that. Dietary GLA reduces inflammation, as it is preferentially converted to DGLA instead of AA. Your body makes small quantities of GLA from LA. It has been used to treat arthritis and some evidence suggests that GLA inhibits the spread of cancers. GLA is found in human and goat milk, organ meats, and borage, primrose, and hemp oils.

DGLA: Dihomo-gamma linoleic acid fights inflammation by preventing the formation of powerful pro-inflammatory prostaglandins, leukotrienes, and thromboxanes that cause factors of inflammation like swelling, pain, fever, and blood clotting. Small amounts of DGLA are present in breast milk and organ meats like liver.

AA: Arachidonic acid is most powerful inflammatory omega-6 fat. Our bodies use it to make prostaglandins and leukotrienes that mobilize our body's inflammatory response, creating the chemical signals that alert our immune cells to attack. In the brain, excess AA makes neurons overly sensitive and excitable. Medicines that fight inflammation and pain like aspirin, ibuprofen, and Celebrex all work by blocking AA. Fats like EPA reduce inflammation by displacing AA from cell membranes.

Omega-7s

CLA: Conjugated linoleic acids are a family of 28 fats made by bacteria in the gut of ruminant animals, like sheep, goats, and cows and found in their milk and meat. They prevent cancer, promote muscle growth, and prevent abdominal fat deposits. Researchers call them body composition modulators, as they reduce body fat while increasing muscle mass. CLA increases blood flow to the brain, protects brain cells from death caused by hyperstimulation called excitotoxicity, and counteracts the effects of the stress hormone cortisol. Grass-fed animals have 300 to 500 percent more CLA than grain-fed ruminants. The most concentrated sources are found in milk and cheese, especially from sheep and goat; and the meat of beef, lamb, goat, and bison.

Monounsaturated

Omega-9s

OLEIC ACID: This is the most abundant fat in the human body and just about everything else: olive oil, beef, fish, almonds, and lard. It is strongly linked to a decreased risk of heart disease, diabetes, and depression. It improves insulin sensitivity. Oleic acid is used by the body to create oleoylethanolamide, which enhances memory, induces fat burning, promotes weight loss, and reduces appetite.

ELAIDIC ACID: Responsible for up to 100,000 heart attacks a year in the United States, this major *trans* fat is found in hydrogenated vegetable oils that make up margarine and other seemingly healthy foods. Elaidic acid is transported to the brain, where it changes the electrical activity of your neurons. It also decreases HDL in your blood while increasing small-dense LDL, which increases your risk of heart disease.

NERVONIC ACID: This is one of the most common fats in myelin, the insulation that drastically increases the speed of signal transmission of neurons and is essential to brain function. Lower levels of this fat are found in children with ADHD. Nervonic acid is linked to a decreased risk of obesity and heart disease. You'll find this fat in salmon, mustard, human breast milk, flaxseed oil, and hemp seeds.

VACCENIC ACID: This fat is made in the stomach of ruminants like cattle and sheep and is found in dairy products. Your body converts it to rumenic acid, a CLA fat that decreases body fat, increases muscle mass, and prevents metabolic syndrome.

Saturated Fats

PALMITIC ACID: Palmitic acid is the most common saturated fat in nature. When your liver converts sugar to fat for storage it produces palmitic acid. It's the main saturated fat in meat and dairy and makes up about 25 percent of the fat in eggs, butter and lard. While it does raises LDL cholesterol, researchers understand today that there are many types of LDL and palmitic acid increases one called light fluffy LDL that appears to actually protect against heart disease.

STEARIC ACID: One of the most common fats in the brain, stearic acid is found in meat and dairy. Stearic acid appears to have neuroprotective effects by activating our neuron's internal antioxidants, which protect brain cells from free radicals. It helps facilitate neurotransmission in the hippocampus, the area of our brain involved in memory, learning, and emotional processing. Levels of this fat are decreased in the brains of patients with Alzheimer's disease. Stearic acid also makes blood less likely to clot, which can reduce the risk of heart attack and stroke, and it has neutral or cholesterol lowering effect.

MARGARIC ACID: This fat, along with pentadecanoic acid, is found in dairy and serves as a biomarker of milk, cheese, and yogurt intake. Used to study the effects of saturated fats on health, the presence of these fats are linked to a decreased risk of a first heart attack.

MYRISTIC ACID: Found in dairy products, human milk, coconut oil, and palm kernel oil, this fat is generally associated with an increased risk of heart disease. However, moderate amounts of dietary myristic acid can improve lipid profiles—decreasing bad LDL and total cholesterol, raising good HDL cholesterol, and preventing the oxidation of fats that contribute to atherosclerosis. Myristic acid also appears to work in synergy with ALA to increase concentrations of the depression-fighting omega-3 fat DHA in cell membranes.

LAURIC ACID: The primary fat in coconut and palm kernel oil, lauric acid also comprises 6 percent of breast milk. It increases total blood cholesterol, but most of the increase is in the form of "good" HDL. Lauric acid can improve insulin function, leading to better blood sugar regulation. It is also known to fight bacteria like *H. pylori*, which cause ulcers, and is being investigated to combat acne.

CAPRIC ACID: This fat is found in goat and sheep's milk. It's also found in few nuts like that of the coconut. It has powerful antibiotic properties and helps our bodies kill bugs like *E. coli*, staph, and gonococci as well as fight off infections from viruses like herpes and HIV.

CAPRYLIC ACID: Found in coconuts and palm oil, as well as in milk, caprylic acid induces neurons to grow new connections and blocks the formation of the inflammatory compound interleukin-8 in the gut. It also has strong antimicrobial and antifungal activity and is needed to activate ghrelin, a hormone that helps regulate hunger.

CAPROIC ACID: Caproic acid is a minor fat found in dairy, especially in goat and sheep milk and cheese. It contributes to the tangy flavor of goat cheese.

BUTYRIC ACID: This is a small, short-chained fatty acid (SCFA) found in butter. While you find small amounts in food, primarily butyric acid is a product of the bacteria in your colon when they digest fiber. This fat supports the health of your gut, as it is the main energy source for the cells that line your large intestine. Butyric acid helps turn off hunger by sending a satiety signal to your brain and also promotes a healthy colon by preventing the growth of cancer cells, cooling off inflammation, and promoting the development of healthy cells. It is known to regulate the expression of over 500 genes.

INTERESTERIFIED FAT: This is a new type of industrially produced fat that has been created by the food industry to replace *trans* fat. While we hear a lot about the dangers of saturated fat, you might be surprised to learn that interesterified fats are saturated. Nothing is known about the long-term safety of this new industrially produced fat. Most people have never heard of interesterified fat, yet it's in many processed food.

Triglycerides

The families of fatty acids—polyunsaturated, monounsaturated, and saturated—are stored and transported in groups of three. They are called *triglycer-ides* because three fatty acids are attached to a molecule called glycerol. When your doctor talks to you about your triglyceride level, he is telling you how much fat is in your blood. In a blood sample, triglycerides float to the top, just like cream separates from milk. Almost all the fat we eat is in the form of triglycerides. That's why all fat is a mix of fats—a combination of, say, a saturated fat, an omega-3 fat, and a monounsaturated fat together form a triglyceride. When your liver converts sugar into fat, you make triglycerides.

Notes

1: What Is Happiness?

3 *Man ought to know:* Hippocrates, *On the Sacred Disease*, 400 B.C.E. Translated by Francis Adams http://classics.mit.edu/Hippocrates/sacred.html

3 *The first detailed anatomical atlas:* Very good illustrated timeline in R. S. Carter et al., *The Human Brain Book*. New York: DK, 2009.

4 *Harvard psychiatrist John Ratey, MD:* John J. Ratey and Albert M. Galaburda, *A User's Guide to the Brain: Perception, Attention, and the Four Theaters of the Brain*, 1st ed. New York: Pantheon Books, 2001.

6 *Our brains have co-evolved:* Stephen C. Cunnane and ebrary Inc., *Survival of the Fattest: The Key to Human Brain Evolution.* Hackensack, NJ: World Scientific, 2005.

6 *running low on iron, a condition:* http://ods.od.nih.gov/factsheets/iron and M. E. Cogswell, L. Kettel-Khan, and U. Ramakrishnan, "Iron Supplement Use among Women in the United States: Science, Policy and Practice," *Journal of Nutrition* 133, no. 6 (2003): 1974S–77S.

7 *leading cause of disability in middle- and high income countries:* S. Moussavi et al., "Depression, Chronic

Diseases, and Decrements in Health: Results from the World Health Surveys." *Lancet* 370 (2007): 851–8.

7 *eating processed foods:* T. N. Akbaraly et al., "Dietary Pattern and Depressive Symptoms in Middle Age," *British Journal of Psychiatry* 195, no. 5 (2009): 408–13.

8 *obese patients who went through weight reduction surgery:* J. Gunstad et al., "Improved Memory Function 12 Weeks after Bariatric Surgery," *Surgery for Obesity and Related Diseases* 7, no. 4 (2011): 465–72.

8 *Rates of obesity and depression:* J. K. Soczynska et al., "Mood Disorders and Obesity: Understanding Inflammation as a Pathophysiological Nexus," *Neuromolecular Medicine* 13, no. 2 (2011): 93–116. See also D. S. Hasin, R. D. Goodwin, F. S. Stinson, and B. F. Grant, "Epidemiology of Major

Depressive Disorder: Results from the National Epidemiologic Survey on Alcoholism and Related Conditions," *Archives of General Psychiatry* 62, no. 10 (2005): 1097–106.

8 *two out of three Americans are overweight:* www.cdc.gov/nchs/fastats/overwt. htm;

www.diabetes.org/diabetes-basics/diabetes-statistics.

8 *Patients with diabetes have much higher rates of depression:* R. J. Anderson, K. E. Freedland, R. E. Clouse, and P. J. Lustman, "The Prevalence of Comorbid Depression in Adults with Diabetes: A Meta-Analysis," *Diabetes Care* 24, no. 6 (2001): 1069–78.

8 *As people with these diseases age:* R. S. McIntyre et al., "Brain Volume Abnormalities and Neurocognitive Deficits in Diabetes Mellitus: Points of Pathophysiological Commonality with Mood Disorders?" *Advances in Therapy* 27, no. 2 (2010): 63–80.

8 *brains of the obese appear sixteen years older:* C. A. Raji et al., "Brain Structure and Obesity," *Human Brain Mapping* 31, no. 3 (2010): 353–64.

9 *The larger the belly size:* R. A. Whitmer et al., "Central Obesity and Increased Risk of Dementia More Than Three Decades Later," *Neurology* 71, no. 14 (2008): 1057–64. See also G. E. Simon et al., "Association Between Obesity and Psychiatric Disorders in the Us Adult Population," *Archives of General Psychiatry* 63, no. 7 (2006): 824–30.

9 *A study of 54,632 women:* M. Lucas et al, "Dietary Intake of N-3 and N-6 Fatty Acids and the Risk of Clinical Depression in Women: A 10-Y Prospective Follow-up Study," *American Journal of Clinical Nutrition* 93, no. 6 (2011): 1337–43.

9 *Research involving 12,059 college graduates:* A. L. Sanchez-Villegas et al., "Dietary Fat Intake and the Risk of Depression: The Sun Project," *PLoS One* 6, no. 1 (2011): e16268.

9 *dietary habits of 4,856 people:* A. R. Wolfe, E. M. Ogbonna, S. Lim, Y. Li, and J. Zhang, "Dietary Linoleic and Oleic Fatty Acids in Relation to Severe Depressed Mood: 10 Years Follow-up of a National Cohort," *Progress in Neuro-Psychopharmacology and Biological Psychiatry* 33, no. 6 (2009): 972–77.

9 *six-week experiment involving children with attention deficit/ hyperactivity disorder:* L. M. Pelsser et al., "Effects of a Restricted Elimination Diet on the Behaviour of Children with Attention-Deficit Hyperactivity Disorder (Inca Study): A Randomised Controlled Trial," *Lancet* 377, no. 9764 (2011): 494–503.

9 *cognitive functions of 280 healthy middle-aged community volunteers:* M. F. Muldoon et al., "Serum Phospholipid Docosahexaenonic Acid Is Associated with Cognitive Functioning During Middle Adulthood," *Journal of Nutrition* 140, no. 4 (2010): 848–53.

11 *information on BDNF and food:* B. Lebrun, B. Bariohay, E. Moyse, and A. Jean, "Brain-Derived Neurotrophic Factor (Bdnf) and Food Intake Regulation: A Minireview," *Autonomic Neuroscience* 126–127 (2006): 30–38.

11 *processed foods high in sugar:* F. N. Jacka et al., "Association of Western and Traditional Diets with Depression and Anxiety in Women," *American Journal of Psychiatry* 167, no. 3 (2010): 305–11.

13 *One study of middle-aged and elderly adults:* I. Bjelland, G. S. Tell, S. E. Vollset, S. Konstantinova, and P. M. Ueland, "Choline in Anxiety and Depression: The Hordaland Health Study," *American Journal of Clinical Nutrition* 90, no. 4 (2009): 1056–60.

2: A Brief History of the Modern American Diet

16 *Southerners in the United States:* M. G. Martin and M. E. Humphreys. "Social Consequence of Disease in the American South, 1900–World War II," *Southern Medical Journal* 99, no. 8 (2006): 862–64.

17 *a food-deficiency disease:* O. P. Kimball, "History of the Prevention of Endemic Goitre," *Bulletin of the World Health Organization* 9, no. 2 (1953): 241–48.

19 *Much of the colonization of the Western Hemisphere:* Sidney Wilfred Mintz, *Sweetness and Power: The Place of Sugar in Modern History.* New York: Penguin, 1986.

21 *the Corn Refiners Association:* www.sweetsurprise.com/news-and-press/press-releases/corn-sugar-fda-petition.

21 *American Sugar Consumption per Year:* Deborah Jean Warner, *Sweet Stuff,* Rowman & Littlefield, 2011; http://www.usda.gov/factbook/chapter2.pdf

22 *Americans drink more than 600 twelve-ounce sodas:* L. R. Vartanian, M. B. Schwartz, and K. D. Brownell, "Effects of Soft Drink Consumption on Nutrition and Health: A Systematic Review and Meta-Analysis," *American Journal of Public Health* 97, no. 4 (April 2007): 667–75.

24 *Together, the brothers-in-law formed:* For an illustrated informative timeline of Proctor and Gamble see: www.pg.com/translations/history_pdf/english_history.pdf.

25 *An issue of* Popular Science *from the era:* H. C. Nixon, "The Rise of the American Cottonseed Oil Industry," *Journal of Political Economy* 38, no. 1 (February 1930): 73–85; at the University of Chicago Press Stable URL: http://www.jstor.org/stable/1823218. Accessed: 24/05/2010 18:06; F. G. Mather, "Waste Products: Cotton-Seed Oil," *Popular Science Monthly,* May 1894, p. 104.

Edwin Kayser, a German chemist: Journal of Industrial Chemical and Engineering Chemistry 9 (December 1917).

28 *Florida's Senator Claude Pepper:* Clarence G. Lasby, *Eisenhower's Heart Attack: How Ike Beat Heart Disease and Held on to the Presidency.* Lawrence: University Press of Kansas, 1997.

28 *281 upper-crust men from Minneapolis:* A. Keys et al., "Coronary Heart Disease among Minnesota Business and Professional Men Followed Fifteen Years," *Circulation* 28 (1963): 381–95.

29 Keys's data were seriously flawed: For a detailed analysis of Keys's work, see G. Taubes, Good Calories, Bad Calories: Fats, Carbs, and the Controversial Science of Diet and Health. New York: Anchor, 2008.

27 *the evidence that animal fats pose this same risk:* P. W. Siri-Tarino, Q. Sun, F. B. Hu, and R. M. Krauss, "Saturated Fat, Carbohydrate, and Cardiovascular Disease," *American Journal of Clinical Nutrition* 91, no. 3 (2010): 502–9; F. B. Hu, J. E. Manson, and W. C. Willett, "Types of Dietary Fat and Risk of Coronary Heart Disease: A Critical Review," *Journal of the American College of Nutrition* 20, no. 1 (2001): 5–19; U. Ravnskov, *Fat and Cholesterol Are Good for You.* GP Publishing, 2009.

29 The Heart Attack Heard 'round America: Lasby, Eisenhower's Heart Attack.

31 consuming trans fats greatly increases: A. L. Sanchez-Villegas, "Dietary Fat Intake and the Risk of Depression: The Sun Project," PLoS One 6, no. 1 (2011): e16268.

31 it allows food manufacturers to claim: fda.gov under "Nutrition Labeling," Questions L1 through L153.

32 they also cross the placenta: J. E. Hunter, "Dietary Trans Fatty Acids: Review of Recent Human Studies and Food Industry Responses," Lipids 41, no. 11 (2006): 967–92.

32 *the more trans fats a pregnant woman eats:* B. Koletzko, "Trans Fatty Acids May Impair Biosynthesis of Long-Chain Polyunsaturates and Growth in Man," *Acta Paediatrica* 81, no. 4 (1992): 302–6.

32 *the more trans fats in a woman's blood:* V. Chajès et al., "Association between Serum Trans-Monounsaturated Fatty Acids and Breast Cancer Risk in the E3n-Epic Study," *American Journal of Epidemiology* 167, no. 11 (2008): 1312–20.

32 *Interestified fats raise blood sugar:* K. C. Hayes and A. Pronczuk, "Replacing Trans Fat: The Argument for Palm Oil with a Cautionary Note on Interesterification," *Journal of the American College of Nutrition* 29, no. 3 Suppl (2010): 253S–84S; K. Sundram, T. Karupaiah, and K. C. Hayes, "Stearic Acid-Rich Interesterified Fat and Trans-Rich Fat Raise the Ldl/Hdl Ratio and Plasma Glucose Relative to Palm Olein in Humans," *Nutrition and Metabolism (London)* 4 (2007): 3.

3: Bad Food, Bad Mood

35 *Type 3 diabetes:* S. M. de la Monteand and J. R. Wands, "Alzheimer's Disease Is Type 3 Diabetes-Evidence Reviewed," *Journal of Diabetes Science and Technology* 2, no. 6 (2008): 1101–13.

34 *increased our sugar intake by 3,000 percent:* Calculated 152 minus 5 divided by 5 times 100 equals 2,940 percent, which we rounded up as these are estimates.

34 *One hundred years later, our sugar consumption:* "Consumption of Sugar," *New York Times,* September 20, 1902.

35 *countries with the highest per capita intake of sugar:* A. N. Westover and L. B. Marangell. "A Cross-National Relationship between Sugar Consumption and Major Depression?" *Depression and Anxiety* 16, no. 3 (2002): 118–20.

35 *Alzheimer's disease "diabetes type 3``:* S. M. de la Monte and J. R. Wands, "Alzheimer's Disease Is Type 3 Diabetes—Evidence Reviewed." *Journal of Diabetes Science and Technology* 2, no. 6 (November 2008): 1101–13.

35 *depression . . . "metabolic syndrome type 2``:* R. S. McIntyre et al., "Should Depressive Syndromes Be Reclassified as 'Metabolic Syndrome Type Ii'?" *Annals of Clinical Psychiatry* 19, no. 4 (October–December 2007): 257–64.

35 *so much sugar shrinks your brain:* R. S. McIntyre et al. "Brain Volume Abnormalities and Neurocognitive Deficits in Diabetes Mellitus: Points of Pathophysiological Commonality with Mood Disorders?" *Advances in Therapy* 27, no. 2 (February 2010): 63–80.

35 *decrease brain-derived neurotrophic factor:* R. Molteni, R. J. Barnard, Z. Ying, C. K. Roberts, and F. Gomez-Pinilla, "A High-Fat, Refined Sugar Diet Reduces Hippocampal Brain-Derived Neurotrophic Factor, Neuronal Plasticity, and Learning," *Neuroscience* 112, no. 4 (2002): 803–14.

35 *smaller hippocampus and amygdala:* Bruehl, H., V. Sweat, A. Tirsi, B. Shah, and A. Convit. "Obese Adolescents with Type 2 Diabetes Mellitus Have Hippocampal and Frontal Lobe Volume Reductions." *Neuroscience & Medicine* 2, no. 1 (2011): 34–42.

37 *simple sugars are addictive:* N. M. Avena, P. Rada, and B. G. Hoebel, "Evidence for Sugar Addiction: Behavioral and Neurochemical Effects of Intermittent, Excessive Sugar Intake," *Neuroscience and Biobehavioral Reviews* 32, no. 1 (2008): 20–39.

38 *pictures activate those same areas:* M. L. Pelchat, A. Johnson, R. Chan, J. Valdez, and J. D. Ragland, "Images of Desire: Food-Craving Activation During fMRI," *NeuroImage* 23, no. 4 (December 2004): 1486–93.

38 *number-one additive in cigarettes is . . . sugar:* Connie Bennett and Stephen Sinatra, *Sugar Shock.* New York: Berkley, 2006, 110-12.

40 *liver converts fructose into triglycerides:* K. L. Stanhope et al. "Consuming Fructose-Sweetened, Not Glucose-Sweetened, Beverages Increases Visceral Adiposity and Lipids and Decreases Insulin Sensitivity in Overweight/Obese Humans," *Journal of Clinical Investigation* 119, no. 5 (May 2009): 1322–34.

40 *fat appears to produce inflammation:* L. Hutley and J. B. Prins. "Fat as an Endocrine Organ: Relationship to the Metabolic Syndrome," *American Journal of the Medical Sciences* 330, no. 6 (December 2005): 280–89.

40 *Fructose boosts production:* K. L. Stanhope et al. "Consuming Fructose-Sweetened, Not Glucose-Sweetened, Beverages Increases Visceral Adiposity . . . "

40 *Fructose shuts down:* A. Shapiro, W. Mu, C. Roncal, K. Y. Cheng, R. J. Johnson, and P. J. Scarpace, "Fructose-Induced Leptin Resistance Exacerbates

Weight Gain in Response to Subsequent High-Fat Feeding," *American Journal of Physiology: Regulatory, Integrative, and Comparative Physiology* 295, no. 5 (November 2008): R1370–75.

40 *Cavities were extremely rare:* Price, Weston A. *Nutrition and Physical Degeneration: A Comparison of Primitive and Modern Diets and Their Effects.* Redlands, Calif.: the author, 1945.

40 *Traditional societies also don't typically have acne:* L. Cordain, S. Lindeberg, M. Hurtado, K. Hill, S. B. Eaton, and J. Brand-Miller. "Acne Vulgaris: A Disease of Western Civilization," *Archives of Dermatology* 138, no. 12 (December 2002): 1584–90. This source also covers the subsequent facts concerning acne and sugar.

41 *most visible signs of glycation are deep wrinkles:* S. F. Ige, R. E. Akhigbe, and A. Akinsanya. "The Role of Hyperglycemia in Skin Wrinkle Formation: Mediation of Advanced Glycation End-Products," *Research Journal of Medical Sciences* 4, no. 5 (2010): 324–29.

41 *AGEs promote inflammation:* R. Singh, A. Barden, T. Mori, and L. Beilin, "Advanced Glycation End-Products: A Review," *Diabetologia* 44, no. 2 (February 2001): 129–46.

41 *at least twenty-four different kinds of cancer:* E. Giovannucci et al., "Diabetes and Cancer: A Consensus Report," *Diabetes Care* 33, no. 7 (July 2010): 1674–85.

42 *the long-term effect of unregulated high blood sugar:* P. J. Beisswenger, "Glycation and Biomarkers of Vascular Complications of Diabetes," *Amino Acids,* November 2, 2010 (epub ahead of print).

43 *greatly increase your risk of depression and heart disease:* A. Sanchez-Villegas et al., "Dietary Fat Intake and the Risk of Depression: The Sun Project," *PLoS One* 6, no. 1 (2011): e16268. See also S. M. Teegala, W. C. Willett, and D. Mozaffarian, "Consumption and Health Effects of Trans Fatty Acids: A Review," *Journal of AOAC International* 92, no. 5 (September–October 2009): 1250.

43 *a proper balance of these fats:* A. R. Wolfe, E. M. Ogbonna, S. Lim, Y. Li, and J. Zhang, "Dietary Linoleic and Oleic Fatty Acids in Relation to Severe Depressed Mood: 10 Years Follow-up of a National Cohort," *Progress in Neuropsychopharmacology and Biological Psychiatry* 33, no. 6 (August 31, 2009): 972–77.

43 *this imbalance more tilted toward omega-6s:* D. Yam, A. Eliraz, and E. M. Berry, "Diet and Disease—the Israeli Paradox: Possible Dangers of a High Omega-6 Polyunsaturated Fatty Acid Diet," *Israel Journal of Medical Sciences* 32, no. 11 (November 1996): 1134–43.

44 *cattle fed an all-grass diet:* N. J. Mann, E. N. Ponnampalam, Y. Yep, and A. J. Sinclair. "Feeding Regimes Affect Fatty Acid Composition in Australian Beef Cattle," *Asia Pacific Journal of Clinical Nutrition* 12 Suppl (2003): S38. See also C. A. Daley, A. Abbott, P. S. Doyle, G. A. Nader, and S. Larson, "A Review of Fatty Acid Profiles and Antioxidant Content in Grass-Fed and Grain-Fed Beef," *Nutrition Journal* 9 (2010): 10.

46 *animals forced to live such miserable lives:* A. L. Schafer, "Role of Nutrition in Reducing Antemortem Stress and Meat Quality Aberrations," *Journal of Animal Science* (2001): 91–101.

46 *Cows are now dosed with anabolic steroids:* http://www.phschool.com/science/science_news/articles/hormones_beef.html

47 *Pigs, too, are fed pharmaceuticals to speed growth:* Fritz Ungemach, "Food, Additives, Series: 53 Ractopamine." http://www.inchem.org/documents/jecfa/jecmono/v53je08.htm#eva. July 7, 2011.

47 *Chicken get fed:* http://www.nytimes.com/2011/06/09/business/09arsenic.html?scp=1&sq=chickens%20arsenic&st=cse.

47 *Russia wouldn't import:* http://www.nytimes.com/2010/01/20/world/europe/20russia.html?scp=1&sq=russia%20chicken%20imports&st=cse.

47 *E. coli . . . didn't become the problem:* L. Horrigan, R. S. Lawrence, and P. Walker, "How Sustainable Agriculture Can Address the Environmental and Human Health Harms of Industrial Agriculture," *Environmental Health Perspectives* 110, no. 5 (May 2002): 445–56.

48 *conventional oranges are injected with dye:* Alissa Hamilton, *Squeezed: What You Don't Know About Orange Juice.* New Haven: Yale University Press, 2009.

49 *produce that's not nearly as healthy:* D. Thomas, "A Study on the Mineral Depletion of the Foods Available to Us as a Nation over the Period 1940 to 1991," *Nutrition and Health* 17, no. 2 (2003): 85–115.

50 *supermarket produce is about 40 percent lower:* V. Worthington, "Effect of Agricultural Methods on Nutritional Quality: A Comparison of Organic with Conventional Crops," *Alternative Therapies in Health and Medicine* 4, no. 1 (January 1998): 58–69.

51 *more than six hundred registered pesticides:* http://www.cdc.gov/nceh/hsb/pesticides/activities.htm.

51 *Researchers at St. Francis Hospital in Indiana:* P. D. Winchester, J. Huskins, and J. Ying, "Agrichemicals in Surface Water and Birth Defects in the United States," *Acta Paediatrica* 98, no. 4 (April 2009): 664–69.

52 *a combination of garlic and fish:* A. J. Adler and B. J. Holub, "Effect of Garlic and Fish-Oil Supplementation on Serum Lipid and Lipoprotein Concentrations in Hypercholesterolemic Men," *American Journal of Clinical Nutrition* 65, no. 2 (Febrary 1997): 445–50.

52 *turmeric . . . being studied:* P. Basnet and N. Skalko-Basnet, "Curcumin: An Anti-Inflammatory Molecule from a Curry Spice on the Path to Cancer Treatment," *Molecules* 16, no. 6 (2011): 4567–98. See also J. Epstein, I. R. Sanderson, and T. T. Macdonald, "Curcumin as a Therapeutic Agent: The Evidence from in Vitro, Animal and Human Studies," *British Journal of Nutrition* 103, no. 11 (June 2010): 1545–57.

53 *Vinegar decreases rice's ability:* M. Sugiyama, A. C. Tang, Y. Wakaki, and W. Koyama, "Glycemic Index of Single and Mixed Meal Foods among Com-

mon Japanese Foods with White Rice as a Reference Food," *European Journal of Clinical Nutrition* 57, no. 6 (June 2003): 743–52.

53 *nutrients work together in the body:* A. Fugh-Berman and F. Kronenberg, "Complementary and Alternative Medicine (Cam) in Reproductive-Age Women: A Review of Randomized Controlled Trials," *Reproductive Toxicology* 17, no. 2 (March–April 2003): 137–52. See also M. Mousain-Bosc, M. Roche, A. Polge, D. Pradal-Prat, J. Rapin, and J. P. Bali, "Improvement of Neurobehavioral Disorders in Children Supplemented with Magnesium-Vitamin B6. I. Attention Deficit Hyperactivity Disorders," *Magnesium Research* 19, no. 1 (March 2006): 46–52.

54 *2010 study in Dallas of 310 food items:* A. Schecter et al., "Perfluorinated Compounds, Polychlorinated Biphenyls, and Organochlorine Pesticide Contamination in Composite Food Samples from Dallas, Texas, USA," *Environmental Health Perspectives* 118, no. 6 (June 2010): 796–802.

55 *Preschool children who eat conventionally:* C. L. Curl, R. A. Fenske, and K. Elgethun, "Organophosphorus Pesticide Exposure of Urban and Suburban Preschool Children with Organic and Conventional Diets," *Environmental Health Perspectives* 111, no. 3 (March 2003): 377–82.

55 *chronic low-grade exposure to pesticides:* C. L. Beseler et al., "Depression and Pesticide Exposures among Private Pesticide Applicators Enrolled in the Agricultural Health Study," *Environmental Health Perspectives* 116, no. 12 (December 2008): 1713–19. See also K. M. Hayden et al., "Occupational Exposure to Pesticides Increases the Risk of Incident AD: The Cache County Study," *Neurology* 74, no. 19 (May 11, 2010): 1524–30.

55 *a study of 33,457 licensed pesticide applicators:* M. P. Montgomery, F. Kamel, T. M. Saldana, M. C. Alavanja, and D. P. Sandler, "Incident Diabetes and Pesticide Exposure among Licensed Pesticide Applicators: Agricultural Health Study, 1993–2003," *American Journal of Epidemiology* 167, no. 10 (May 15 2008): 1235–46.

4: Good Food, Good Mood

Vitamin B₁₂

Bradford, G. S., and C. T. Taylor, "Omeprazole and Vitamin B12 Deficiency," *Annals of Pharmacotherapy* 33, no. 5 (May 1999): 641–3.

Coppen, A., and C. Bolander-Gouaille, "Treatment of Depression: Time to Consider Folic Acid and Vitamin B12," *Journal of Psychopharmacology* 19, no. 1 (January 2005): 59–65.

Garcia-Manzanares, A., and A. J. Lucendo, "Nutritional and Dietary Aspects of Celiac Disease," *Nutrition in Clinical Practice* 26, no. 2 (April 2011): 163–73.

Li, D, "Chemistry Behind Vegetarianism," *Journal of Agricultural and Food Chemistry* 59, no. 3 (February 9, 2011): 777–84.

Selhub, J., A. Troen, and I. H. Rosenberg, "B Vitamins and the Aging Brain," *Nutrition Reviews* 68 Suppl. 2 (December 2010): S112–8.

Iodine

Costa, L. G., G. Giordano, S. Tagliaferri, A. Caglieri, and A. Mutti, "Polybrominated Diphenyl Ether (Pbde) Flame Retardants: Environmental Contamination, Human Body Burden and Potential Adverse Health Effects," *Acta Biomedica* 79, no. 3 (December 2008): 172–83.

Hollowell, J. G., et al., "Iodine Nutrition in the United States. Trends and Public Health Implications: Iodine Excretion Data from National Health and Nutrition Examination Surveys I and Iii (1971–1974 and 1988–1994)," *Journal of Clinical Endocrinology and Metabolism* 83, no. 10 (October 1998): 3401–8.

Laurberg, P., et al., "Iodine Intake as a Determinant of Thyroid Disorders in Populations," *Best Practices and Research: Clinical Endocrinology and Metabolism* 24, no. 1 (February 2010): 13–27.

Pavelka, S., "Metabolism of Bromide and Its Interference with the Metabolism of Iodine," *Physiological Research* 53, Suppl. 1 (2004): S81–90.

Magnesium

Eby, G. A., 3rd, and K. L. Eby, "Magnesium for Treatment-Resistant Depression: A Review and Hypothesis," *Medical Hypotheses* 74, no. 4 (April 2010): 649–60.

Ismail, Y., and A. A. Ismail, "The Underestimated Problem of Using Serum Magnesium Measurements to Exclude Magnesium Deficiency in Adults; a Health Warning Is Needed for 'Normal' Results," *Clinical Chemistry and Laboratory* 48, no. 3 (March 2010): 323–27.

Jacka, F. N., S. Overland, R. Stewart, G. S. Tell, I. Bjelland, and A. Mykletun, "Association Between Magnesium Intake and Depression and Anxiety in Community-Dwelling Adults: The Hordaland Health Study," *Australian and New Zealand Journal of Psychiatry* 43, no. 1 (January 2009): 45–52.

Slutsky, I., N. et al., "Enhancement of Learning and Memory by Elevating Brain Magnesium," *Neuron* 65, no. 2 (January 28, 2010): 165–77.

Cholesterol

Aijanseppa, S., et al., "Serum Cholesterol and Depressive Symptoms in Elderly Finnish Men," *International Journal of Geriatric Psychiatry* 17, no. 7 (July 2002): 629–34.

Djousse, L., and J. M. Gaziano, "Egg Consumption in Relation to Cardiovascular Disease and Mortality: The Physicians' Health Study," *American Journal of Clinical Nutrition* 87, no. 4 (April 2008): 964–69.

Egert, S., M. Kratz, F. Kannenberg, M. Fobker, and U. Wahrburg, "Effects of High-Fat and Low-Fat Diets Rich in Monounsaturated Fatty Acids on Serum Lipids, Ldl Size and Indices of Lipid Peroxidation in Healthy Non-Obese Men and Women When Consumed under Controlled Conditions," *European Journal of Clinical Nutrition* 50, no. 1 (Feb 2011): 71–79.

Henderson, V. W., J. R. Guthrie, and L. Dennerstein, "Serum Lipids and Memory in a Population Based Cohort of Middle-Age Women," *Journal of Neurology, Neurosurgery, and Psychiatry* 74, no. 11 (November 2003): 1530–35.

Hu, F. B., et al., "A Prospective Study of Egg Consumption and Risk of Cardiovascular Disease in Men and Women," *Journal of the American Medical Association* 281, no. 15 (April 21, 1999): 1387–94.

Hunter, J. E., "Dietary Trans Fatty Acids: Review of Recent Human Studies and Food Industry Responses," *Lipids* 41, no. 11 (November 2006): 967–92.

Lamarche, B., et al., "Small, Dense Low-Density Lipoprotein Particles as a Predictor of the Risk of Ischemic Heart Disease in Men. Prospective Results from the Quebec Cardiovascular Study," *Circulation* 95, no. 1 (January 7, 1997): 69–75.

Lutjohann, D., "Brain Cholesterol and Suicidal Behaviour," *International Journal of Neuropsychopharmacology* 10, no. 2 (April 2007): 153–57.

Mielke, M. M., et al., "High Total Cholesterol Levels in Late Life Associated with a Reduced Risk of Dementia," *Neurology* 64, no. 10 (May 24, 2005): 1689–95.

Mozaffarian, D., M. B. Katan, A. Ascherio, M. J. Stampfer, and W. C. Willett, "Trans Fatty Acids and Cardiovascular Disease," *New England Journal of Medicine* 354, no. 15 (April 13, 2006): 1601–13.

Papakostas, G. I., D. Ongur, D. V. Iosifescu, D. Mischoulon, and M. Fava, "Cholesterol in Mood and Anxiety Disorders: Review of the Literature and New Hypotheses," *European Neuropsychopharmacology* 14, no. 2 (March 2004): 135–42.

Schreurs, B. G., "The Effects of Cholesterol on Learning and Memory," *Neuroscience and Biobehavioral Reviews* 34, no. 8 (July 2010): 1366–79.

Shrivastava, S., T. J. Pucadyil, Y. D. Paila, S. Ganguly, and A. Chattopadhyay, "Chronic Cholesterol Depletion Using Statin Impairs the Function and Dynamics of Human Serotonin(1a) Receptors," *Biochemistry* 49, no. 26 (July 6, 2010): 5426–35.

West, R., et al., "Better Memory Functioning Associated with Higher Total and Low-Density Lipoprotein Cholesterol Levels in Very Elderly Subjects without the Apolipoprotein E4 Allele," *American Journal of Geriatric Psychiatry* 16, no. 9 (September 2008): 781–85.

Vitamin D

Barnard, K., and C. Colon-Emeric, "Extraskeletal Effects of Vitamin D in Older Adults: Cardiovascular Disease, Mortality, Mood, and Cognition," *American Journal of Geriatric Pharmacotherapy* 8, no. 1 (February 2010): 4–33.

Cannell, J. J., et al., "Epidemic Influenza and Vitamin D," *Epidemiology and Infection* 134, no. 6 (December 2006): 1129–40.

Clausen, I., J. Jakobsen, T. Leth, and L. Ovesen, "Vitamin D$_3$ and 25-Hydroxyvitamin D$_3$ in Raw and Cooked Pork Cuts," *Journal of Food Composition and Analysis* 16, no. 5 (October 2003): 575–85.

Holick, M. F., and T. C. Chen, "Vitamin D Deficiency: A Worldwide Problem with Health Consequences," *American Journal of Clinical Nutrition* 87, no. 4 (April 2008): 1080S–6S.

Holick, M. F., "Vitamin D Deficiency," *New England Journal of Medicine* 357, no. 3 (July 19, 2007): 266–81.

McCann, J. C., and B. N. Ames, "Is There Convincing Biological or Behavioral Evidence Linking Vitamin D Deficiency to Brain Dysfunction?" *FASEB Journal* 22, no. 4 (April 2008): 982–1001.

Wagner, C. L., T. C. Hulsey, D. Fanning, M. Ebeling, and B. W. Hollis, "High-Dose Vitamin D3 Supplementation in a Cohort of Breastfeeding Mothers and Their Infants: A 6-Month Follow-up Pilot Study," *Breastfeeding Medicine Journal* 1, no. 2 (Summer 2006): 59–70.

Wilkins, C. H., Y. I. Sheline, C. M. Roe, S. J. Birge, and J. C. Morris, "Vitamin D Deficiency Is Associated with Low Mood and Worse Cognitive Performance in Older Adults," *American Journal of Geriatric Psychiatry* 14, no. 12 (December 2006): 1032–40.

Calcium

Finkbeiner, S., "Calcium Regulation of the Brain-Derived Neurotrophic Factor Gene," *Cellular and Molecular Life Sciences* 57, no. 3 (March 2000): 394–401.

Jones, E. G., "Calcium Channels in Higher-Level Brain Function," *Proceedings of the National Academy of Sciences of the United States of America* 104, no. 46 (November 13, 2007): 17903–4.

Mangano, K. M., S. J. Walsh, K. L. Insogna, A. M. Kenny, and J. E. Kerstetter, "Calcium Intake in the United States from Dietary and Supplemental Sources across Adult Age Groups: New Estimates from the National Health and Nutrition Examination Survey 2003–2006," *Journal of the American Dietetic Association* 111, no. 5 (May 2011): 687–95.

Thys-Jacobs, S., "Micronutrients and the Premenstrual Syndrome: The Case for Calcium," *Journal of the American College of Nutrition* 19, no. 2 (April 2000): 220–27.

Tsialtas, D., et al., "Stented Versus Stentless Bioprostheses in Aortic Valve Stenosis: Effect on Left Ventricular Remodelling," *Heart Surgery Forum* 10, no. 3 (2007): E205–10.

Fiber

Anderson, J. W., et al., "Health Benefits of Dietary Fiber," *Nutrition Reviews* 67, no. 4 (April 2009): 188–205.

Galland, L., "Diet and Inflammation," *Nutrition in Clinical Practice* 25, no. 6 (December 2010): 634–40.

Liu, S., et al., "Relation between Changes in Intakes of Dietary Fiber and Grain Products and Changes in Weight and Development of Obesity among Middle-Aged Women," *American Journal of Clinical Nutrition* 78, no. 5 (Nov 2003): 920–27.

Logan, A. C., "Dietary Fiber, Mood, and Behavior," *Nutrition* 22, no. 2 (February 2006): 213–4; author reply 15.

Ma, Y., et al., "Association Between Dietary Fiber and Markers of Systemic Inflammation in the Women's Health Initiative Observational Study," *Nutrition* 24, no. 10 (Oct 2008): 941–49.

Zhang, J., Y. Li, and M. E. Torres, "How Does a Suicide Attempter Eat Differently from Others? Comparison of Macronutrient Intakes," *Nutrition* 21, no. 6 (June 2005): 711–17.

Folate

Coppen, A., and C. Bolander-Gouaille, "Treatment of Depression: Time to Consider Folic Acid and Vitamin B12," *Journal of Psychopharmacology* 19, no. 1 (January 2005): 59–65.

Das, U. N., "Folic Acid and Polyunsaturated Fatty Acids Improve Cognitive Function and Prevent Depression, Dementia, and Alzheimer's Disease—but How and Why?" *Prostaglandins, Leukotrienes, and Essential Fatty Acids* 78, no. 1 (January 2008): 11–9.

Konings, E. J., et al., "Intestinal Absorption of Different Types of Folate in Healthy Subjects with an Ileostomy," *British Journal of Nutrition* 88, no. 3 (September 2002): 235–42.

Malouf, R., and J. Grimley Evans, "Folic Acid with or Without Vitamin B12 for the Prevention and Treatment of Healthy Elderly and Demented People," *Cochrane Database of Systematic Reviews*, no. 4 (2008): CD004514.

McNulty, H., and K. Pentieva, "Folate Bioavailability," *Proceedings of the Nutrition Society* 63, no. 4 (November 2004): 529–36.

Ramos, M. I., et al., "Low Folate Status Is Associated with Impaired Cognitive Function and Dementia in the Sacramento Area Latino Study on Aging," *American Journal of Clinical Nutrition* 82, no. 6 (December 2005): 1346–52.

Williams, E., B. Stewart-Knox, C. McConville, I. Bradbury, N. C. Armstrong, and H. McNulty, "Folate Status and Mood: Is There a Relationship?" *Public Health Nutrition* 11, no. 2 (February 2008): 118–23.

Vitamin A

Bremner, J. D., and P. McCaffery, "The Neurobiology of Retinoic Acid in Affective Disorders," *Progress in Neuro-Psychopharmacology and Biological Psychiatry* 32, no. 2 (February 15, 2008): 315–31.

Lane, M. A., and S. J. Bailey, "Role of Retinoid Signalling in the Adult Brain," *Progress in Neurobiology* 75, no. 4 (March 2005): 275–93.

Tanumihardjo, S. A., "Factors Influencing the Conversion of Carotenoids to Retinol: Bioavailability to Bioconversion to Bioefficacy," *International Journal for Vitamin and Nutrition Research* 72, no. 1 (January 2002): 40–45.

Tanumihardjo, S. A., "Vitamin A: Biomarkers of Nutrition for Development," *American Journal of Clinical Nutrition* (June 29, 2011).

Omega-3s

Arterburn, L. M., E. B. Hall, and H. Oken, "Distribution, Interconversion, and Dose Response of N-3 Fatty Acids in Humans," *American Journal of Clinical Nutrition* 83, no. 6, Suppl. (June 2006): 1467S-76S.

Bourre, J. M. "Effects of Nutrients (in Food) on the Structure and Function of the Nervous System: Update on Dietary Requirements for Brain. Part 2 : Macronutrients," *Journal of Nutrition, Health and Aging* 10, no. 5 (September–October 2006): 386–99.

Brenna, J. T., N. Salem, Jr., A. J. Sinclair, and S. C. Cunnane, "Alpha-Linolenic Acid Supplementation and Conversion to N-3 Long-Chain Polyunsaturated Fatty Acids in Humans," *Prostaglandins, Leukotrienes, and Essential Fatty Acids* 80, no. 2–3 (February–March 2009): 85–91.

Conklin, S. M., et al., "Long-Chain Omega-3 Fatty Acid Intake Is Associated Positively with Corticolimbic Gray Matter Volume in Healthy Adults," *Neuroscience Letters* 421, no. 3 (June 29, 2007): 209–12.

Stevens, L. J., S. S. Zentall, M. L. Abate, T. Kuczek, and J. R. Burgess, "Omega-3 Fatty Acids in Boys with Behavior, Learning, and Health Problems," *Physiology and Behavior* 59, no. 4–5 (April–May 1996): 915–20.

Sublette, M. E., J. R. Hibbeln, H. Galfalvy, M. A. Oquendo, and J. J. Mann, "Omega-3 Polyunsaturated Essential Fatty Acid Status as a Predictor of Future Suicide Risk," *American Journal of Psychiatry* 163, no. 6 (June 2006): 1100–2.

Wu, A., Z. Ying, and F. Gomez-Pinilla, "Docosahexaenoic Acid Dietary Supplementation Enhances the Effects of Exercise on Synaptic Plasticity and Cognition," *Neuroscience* 155, no. 3 (August 26, 2008): 751–59.

Vitamin E

Aggarwal, B. B., C. Sundaram, S. Prasad, and R. Kannappan, "Tocotrienols, the Vitamin E of the 21st Century: Its Potential against Cancer and Other Chronic Diseases," *Biochemical Pharmacology* 80, no. 11 (December 1, 2010): 1613–31.

Jiang, Q., S. Christen, M. K. Shigenaga, and B. N. Ames, "Gamma-Tocopherol, the Major Form of Vitamin E in the Us Diet, Deserves More Attention," *American Journal of Clinical Nutrition* 74, no. 6 (December 2001): 714–22.

Khanna, S., et al., "Molecular Basis of Vitamin E Action: Tocotrienol Modulates 12-Lipoxygenase, a Key Mediator of Glutamate-Induced Neurodegeneration," *Journal of Biological Chemistry* 278, no. 44 (October 31, 2003): 43508–15.

Maras, J. E., et al., "Intake of Alpha-Tocopherol Is Limited among Us Adults," *Journal of the American Dietetic Association* 104, no. 4 (April 2004): 567–75.

Morris, M. C., et al., "Relation of the Tocopherol Forms to Incident Alzheimer Disease and to Cognitive Change," *American Journal of Clinical Nutrition* 81, no. 2 (February 2005): 508–14.

Owen, A. J., M. J. Batterham, Y. C. Probst, B. F. Grenyer, and L. C. Tapsell, "Low Plasma Vitamin E Levels in Major Depression: Diet or Disease?" *European Journal of Clinical Nutrition* 59, no. 2 (February 2005): 304–6.

Sen, C. K., S. Khanna, and S. Roy, "Tocotrienol: The Natural Vitamin E to Defend the Nervous System?" *Annals of the New York Academy of Science* 1031 (December 2004): 127–42.

Iron

Beard, J., "Iron Deficiency Alters Brain Development and Functioning," *Journal of Nutrition* 133, no. 5, Suppl. 1 (May 2003): 1468S–72S.

Salvador, G. A., "Iron in Neuronal Function and Dysfunction," *Biofactors* 36, no. 2 (March–April 2010): 103–10.

Youdim, M. B., "Brain Iron Deficiency and Excess; Cognitive Impairment and Neurodegeneration with Involvement of Striatum and Hippocampus," *Neurotoxicity Research* 14, no. 1 (August 2008): 45–56.

5: Food for Thought

86 *scientists at the University of California:* O. Quehenberger et al. "Lipidomics Reveals a Remarkable Diversity of Lipids in Human Plasma," *Journal of Lipid Research* 51, no. 11 (November 2010): 3299–305.

87 *CLA is the only fat recognized:* M. A. McGuire and M. K. McGuire, "Conjugated Linoleic Acid (CLA): A Ruminant Fatty Acid with Beneficial Effects on Human Health," *Proceedings of the American Society of Animal Science,* 1999 [online publication].

87 *CLA . . . protects brain cells:* W. T. Hunt, A. Kamboj, H. D. Anderson, and C. M. Anderson, "Protection of Cortical Neurons from Excitotoxicity by Conjugated Linoleic Acid," *Journal of Neurochemistry* 115, no. 1 (October 2010): 123–30.

87 *Grass-fed animals have 300 to 500 percent:* T. R. Dhiman, G. R. Anand, L. D. Satter, and M. W. Pariza, "Conjugated Linoleic Acid Content of Milk from Cows Fed Different Diets," *Journal of Dairy Science* 82, no. 10 (October 1999): 2146–56.

87 *CLA prevents cancer:* Heinze, V. M., and A. B. Actis. "Dietary Conjugated Linoleic Acid and Long-Chain N-3 Fatty Acids in Mammary and Prostate Cancer Protection: A Review." *Int J Food Sci Nutr* (2011).

87 *abdominal fat deposits:* J. M. Gaullier et al., "Supplementation with Conjugated Linoleic Acid for 24 Months Is Well Tolerated by and Reduces Body Fat Mass in Healthy, Overweight Humans," *Journal of Nutrition* 135, no. 4 (April 2005): 778–84.

87 *Researchers call CLA:* Y. Wangand P. J. Jones, "Dietary Conjugated Linoleic Acid and Body Composition," *American Journal of Clinical Nutrition* 79, no. 6, Suppl. (June 2004): 1153S–58S.

88 *consumption of dairy is linked:* S. Aslibekyan, H. Campos, and A. Baylin, "Biomarkers of Dairy Intake and the Risk of Heart Disease," *Nutrition, Metabolism, and Cardiovascular Diseases*, May 4, 2011. See also E. Sonestedt et al., "Dairy Products and Its Association with Incidence of Cardiovascular Disease: The Malmo Diet and Cancer Cohort," *European Journal of Epidemiology*, June 10, 2011; and V. S. Malik et al., "Adolescent Dairy Product Consumption and Risk of Type 2 Diabetes in Middle-Aged Women," *American Journal of Clinical Nutrition*, July 13, 2011.

92 *DIM can also stop cancer cells:* J. V. Higdon, B. Delage, D. E. Williams, and R. H. Dashwood, "Cruciferous Vegetables and Human Cancer Risk: Epidemiologic Evidence and Mechanistic Basis," *Pharmacological Research* 55, no. 3 (March 2007): 224–36.

93 *flavonoid family of phytonutrients:* E. J. Choi and W. S. Ahn, "Neuroprotective Effects of Chronic Hesperetin Administration in Mice," *Archives of Pharmacal Research* 31, no. 11 (November 2008): 1457–62; H. J. Heo et al., "Effect of Antioxidant Flavanone, Naringenin, from Citrus Junoson Neuroprotection," *Journal of Agricultural and Food Chemistry* 52, no. 6 (March 24, 2004): 1520–55.

93 *flavonoids reduce inflammation:* J. P. Spencer, "The Interactions of Flavonoids within Neuronal Signalling Pathways," *Genes & Nutrition* 2, no. 3 (December 2007): 257–73.

93 *Flavonoids also enhance mental functioning:* J. Terao, Y. Kawai, and K. Murota, "Vegetable Flavonoids and Cardiovascular Disease," *Asia Pacific Journal of Clinical Nutrition* 17 Suppl. 1 (2008): 291–93.

93 *Naringenin . . . blocks the enzyme acetylcholinesterase:* H. J. Heo et al., "Naringenin from Citrus Junos Has an Inhibitory Effect on Acetylcholinesterase

and a Mitigating Effect on Amnesia," *Dementia and Geriatric Cognitive Disorders* 17, no. 3 (2004): 151–57.

93 *Hesperetin protects neurons:* S. L. Hwang and G. C. Yen, "Neuroprotective Effects of the Citrus Flavanones against H2o2-Induced Cytotoxicity in Pc12 Cells," *Journal of Agricultural and Food Chemistry* 56, no. 3 (February 13, 2008): 859–64.

94 *hesperetin also binds to our opioid receptors:* L. M. Loscalzo, C. Wasowski, A. C. Paladini, and M. Marder, "Opioid Receptors Are Involved in the Sedative and Antinociceptive Effects of Hesperidin as Well as in Its Potentiation with Benzodiazepines," *European Journal of Pharmacology* 580, no. 3 (February 12, 2008): 306–13.

94 *limonoids . . . keep your brain cells healthy:* A. Roy and S. Saraf, "Limonoids: Overview of Significant Bioactive Triterpenes Distributed in Plants Kingdom," *Biological & Pharmaceutical Bulletin* 29, no. 2 (February 2006): 191–201.

96 *anthocyanins that protect the neurons:* J. A. Joseph, B. Shukitt-Hale, and L. M. Willis, "Grape Juice, Berries, and Walnuts Affect Brain Aging and Behavior," *Journal of Nutrition* 139, no. 9 (September 2009): 1813S–7S.

96 *blueberries . . . improve spatial memory:* C. M. Williams et al., "Blueberry-Induced Changes in Spatial Working Memory Correlate with Changes in Hippocampal Creb Phosphorylation and Brain-Derived Neurotrophic Factor (Bdnf) Levels," *Free Radical Biology & Medicine* 45, no. 3 (August 1, 2008): 295–305.

96 *strawberries are loaded with fisetin:* P. Maher, R. Dargusch, J. L. Ehren, S. Okada, K. Sharma, and D. Schubert, "Fisetin Lowers Methylglyoxal Dependent Protein Glycation and Limits the Complications of Diabetes," *PLoS One* 6, no. 6 (2011): e21226. See also P. Maher, T. Akaishi, and K. Abe, "Flavonoid Fisetin Promotes Erk-Dependent Long-Term Potentiation and Enhances Memory," *Proceedings of the National Academy of Sciences of the United States of America* 103, no. 44 (October 31, 2006): 16568–73.

96 *cranberries contain a unique phytochemical called proanthocyanidin:* A. B. Howell, "Cranberry Proanthocyanidins and the Maintenance of Urinary Tract Health," *Critical Reviews in Food Science and Nutrition* 42, no. 3 Suppl. (2002): 273–78.

97 *Kids who get more of these fatty acids:* C. R. Gale et al., "Oily Fish Intake During Pregnancy—Association with Lower Hyperactivity but Not with Higher Full-Scale IQ in Offspring," *Journal of Child Psychology and Psychiatry, and Allied Disciplines* 49, no. 10 (October 2008): 1061–68. See also J. R. Hibbeln et al., "Maternal Seafood Consumption in Pregnancy and Neurodevelopmental Outcomes in Childhood (Alspac Study): An Observational Cohort Study," *Lancet* 369, no. 9561 (February 17, 2007): 578–85.

97 *the omega-3s in anchovies:* R. De Caterina, "N-3 Fatty Acids in Cardiovascular Disease," *New England Journal of Medicine* 364, no. 25 (June 23, 2011): 2439–50.

97 *coenzyme Q10 . . . slow down the progression of Parkinson's disease:* C. W. Shults et al., "Effects of Coenzyme Q10 in Early Parkinson Disease: Evidence of Slowing of the Functional Decline," *Archives of Neurology* 59, no. 10 (October 2002): 1541–50.

6: Food for Energy

100 *many cancerous cells have low levels of methylation:* Y. Watanabe and M. Maekawa, "Methylation of DNA in Cancer," *Advances in Clinical Chemistry* 52 (2010): 145–67.

101 *red pigments called carotenoids:* H. Tapiero, D. M. Townsend, and K. D. Tew, "The Role of Carotenoids in the Prevention of Human Pathologies," *Biomedicine & Pharmacotherapy* 58, no. 2 (March 2004): 100–10. See also P. Di Mascio, M. E. Murphy, and H. Sies, "Antioxidant Defense Systems: The Role of Carotenoids, Tocopherols, and Thiols," *American Journal of Clinical Nutrition* 53, no. 1 Suppl. (January 1991): 194S–200S.

101 *Heating them turbocharges their sulforaphane content:* N. V. Matusheski, J. A. Juvik, and E. H. Jeffery, "Heating Decreases Epithiospecifier Protein Activity and Increases Sulforaphane Formation in Broccoli," *Phytochemistry* 65, no. 9 (May 2004): 1273–81.

101 *Sulforaphanes ignite the liver's detoxification system:* J. D. Clarke, R. H. Dashwood, and E. Ho, "Multi-Targeted Prevention of Cancer by Sulforaphane," *Cancer Letters* 269, no. 2 (October 8, 2008): 291–304.

102 *In the brain it blocks the action of a neurotransmitter:* Z. Huang et al., "Adenosine A2a, but Not A1, Receptors Mediate the Arousal Effect of Caffeine," *Nature Neuroscience* 8, no. 7 (July 2005): 858–59. See also M. Solinas et al., "Caffeine Induces Dopamine and Glutamate Release in the Shell of the Nucleus Accumbens," *The Journal of Neuroscience* 22, no. 15 (August 1, 2002): 6321–24.

102 *a cup of coffee has more antioxidant phytonutrients:* B. L. Halvorsen et al., "Content of Redox-Active Compounds (Ie, Antioxidants) in Foods Consumed in the United States," *American Journal of Clinical Nutrition* 84, no. 1 (July 2006): 95–135.

102 *norharman and Harman:* T. Herraiz and C. Chaparro, "Human Monoamine Oxidase Enzyme Inhibition by Coffee and Beta-Carbolines Norharman and Harman Isolated from Coffee," *Life Sciences* 78, no. 8 (January 18, 2006): 795–A802.

103 *A study in Finland followed 1,409 people:* M. H. Eskelinen and M. Kivipelto, "Caffeine as a Protective Factor in Dementia and Alzheimer's Disease," *Journal of Alzheimer's Disease* 20 Suppl. 1 (2010): S167–74.

103 *A massive study published in the Archives of Internal Medicine:* R. Huxley et al., "Coffee, Decaffeinated Coffee, and Tea Consumption in Relation to Incident Type 2 Diabetes Mellitus: A Systematic Review with Meta-Analysis," *Archives of Internal Medicine* 169, no. 22 (December 14, 2009): 2053–63.

103 *flavonols like epicatechin:* J. P. Spencer, "Beyond Antioxidants: The Cellular and Molecular Interactions of Flavonoids and How These Underpin Their Actions on the Brain," *Proceedings of the Nutrition Society* 69, no. 2 (May 2010): 244–60. See also N. D. Fisher, F. A. Sorond, and N. K. Hollenberg, "Cocoa Flavanols and Brain Perfusion," *Journal of Cardiovascular Pharmacology* 47 Suppl. 2 (2006): S210–4.

103 *study from the* Journal of Psychopharmacology: A. B. Scholey et al., "Consumption of Cocoa Flavanols Results in Acute Improvements in Mood and Cognitive Performance During Sustained Mental Effort," *Journal of Psychopharmacology* 24, no. 10 (October 2010): 1505–14.

104 *It even makes cells more sensitive to insulin:* D. Grassi, C. Lippi, S. Necozione, G. Desideri, and C. Ferri, "Short-Term Administration of Dark Chocolate Is Followed by a Significant Increase in Insulin Sensitivity and a Decrease in Blood Pressure in Healthy Persons," *American Journal of Clinical Nutrition* 81, no. 3 (March 2005): 611–4. See also S. Almoosawi, L. Fyfe, C. Ho, and E. Al-Dujaili, "The Effect of Polyphenol-Rich Dark Chocolate on Fasting Capillary Whole Blood Glucose, Total Cholesterol, Blood Pressure and Glucocorticoids in Healthy Overweight and Obese Subjects," *British Journal of Nutrition* 103, no. 6 (March 2010): 842–50.

105 *various forms of vitamin E:* C. K. Sen, S. Khanna, and S. Roy, "Tocotrienol: The Natural Vitamin E to Defend the Nervous System?" *Annals of the New York Academy of Science* 1031 (December 2004): 127–42.

105 *patients with depression often have low levels of vitamin E:* A. J. Owen, M. J. Batterham, Y. C. Probst, B. F. Grenyer, and L. C. Tapsell, "Low Plasma Vitamin E Levels in Major Depression: Diet or Disease?" *European Journal of Clinical Nutrition* 59, no. 2 (February 2005): 304–6. See also M. Maes et al., "Lower Serum Vitamin E Concentrations in Major Depression. Another Marker of Lowered Antioxidant Defenses in That Illness," *Journal of Affective Disorders* 58, no. 3 (June 2000): 241–46.

106 *Adventists found that those who consumed nuts:* G. E. Fraser, J. Sabate, W. L. Beeson, and T. M. Strahan, "A Possible Protective Effect of Nut Consumption on Risk of Coronary Heart Disease. The Adventist Health Study," *Archives of Internal Medicine* 152, no. 7 (July 1992): 1416–24.

106 *the USDA tested the antioxidant capacity of 147 of the most commonly eaten plant foods:* X. Wu et al., "Lipophilic and Hydrophilic Antioxidant Capacities of Common Foods in the United States," *Journal of Agricultural and Food Chemistry* 52, no. 12 (June 16, 2004): 4026–37.

106 *seeds' phytates:* A. Rose and A. Adams, *Rebuild from Depression: A Nutrient Guide Including Depression in Pregnancy and Postpartum.* California Hot Springs, Calif.: Purple Oak Press, 2009. See also I. Lestienne, "Effects of Soaking Whole Cereal and Legume Seeds on Iron, Zinc, and Phytate Contents," *Food Chemistry* 89, no. 3 (2005): 421–25.

107 *the International Potato Center in Lima:* http://www.cipotato.org

107 *the third most consumed plant on the planet:* M. E. Camire, S. Kubow, and D. J. Donnelly, "Potatoes and Human Health," *Critical Reviews in Food Science and Nutrition* 49, no. 10 (November 2009): 823–40.

107 *One particularly rare group of molecules in potatoes:* A. J. Parr, F. A. Mellon, I. J. Colquhoun, and H. V. Davies, "Dihydrocaffeoyl Polyamines (Kukoamine and Allies) in Potato (Solanum Tuberosum) Tubers Detected During Metabolite Profiling," *Journal of Agricultural and Food Chemistry* 53, no. 13 (June 29, 2005): 5461–66.

108 *Frying potatoes at high heat:* A. Becalski et al., "Acrylamide in French Fries: Influence of Free Amino Acids and Sugars," *Journal of Agricultural and Food Chemistry* 52, no. 12 (June 16, 2004): 3801–6.

108 *Small potatoes have three times:* A. Goyer and D. A. Navarre, "Folate Is Higher in Developmentally Younger Potato Tubers," *Journal of the Science of Food and Agriculture* 89, no. 4 (2009): 579–83.

7: Food for Good Mood

112 *When it comes to incredible feats of endurance:* D. Maillet and J. M. Weber, "Performance-Enhancing Role of Dietary Fatty Acids in a Long-Distance Migrant Shorebird: The Semipalmated Sandpiper," *Journal of Experimental Biology* 209, no. 14 (July 2006): 2686–95.

113 *When studies compare the mood disorders in different countries*: S. Noaghiul and J. R. Hibbeln, "Cross-National Comparisons of Seafood Consumption and Rates of Bipolar Disorders," *American Journal of Psychiatry* 160, no. 12 (December 2003): 2222–27. See also J. R. Hibbeln, "Seafood Consumption, the DHA Content of Mothers' Milk and Prevalence Rates of Postpartum Depression: A Cross-National, Ecological Analysis," *Journal of Affective Disorders* 69, no. 1–3 (May 2002): 15–29.

113 *depression has increased about twentyfold:* G. L. Klerman and M. M. Weissman, "Increasing Rates of Depression," *Journal of the American Medical Association* 261, no. 15 (April 21, 1989): 2229–35. See also "The Changing Rate of Major Depression. Cross-National Comparisons. Cross-National Collaborative Group," *Journal of the American Medical Association* 268, no. 21 (December 2, 1992): 3098–105.

113 *Patients diagnosed with depression:* R. Edwards, M. Peet, J. Shay, and D. Horrobin, "Omega-3 Polyunsaturated Fatty Acid Levels in the Diet and in Red Blood Cell Membranes of Depressed Patients," *Journal of Affective Disorders* 48, no. 2–3 (March 1998): 149–55.

113 *A study of one hundred patients in China:* M. Huan et al., "Suicide Attempt and N-3 Fatty Acid Levels in Red Blood Cells: A Case Control Study in China," *Biological Psychiatry* 56, no. 7 (October 1, 2004): 490–96.

113 *People who commit suicide eat less fish:* M. E. Sublette, J. R. Hibbeln, H. Galfalvy, M. A. Oquendo, and J. J. Mann, "Omega-3 Polyunsaturated

Essential Fatty Acid Status as a Predictor of Future Suicide Risk," *American Journal of Psychiatry* 163, no. 6 (June 2006): 1100–2.

113 *Young boys with lower levels of omega-3s:* L. J. Stevens, S. S. Zentall, M. L. Abate, T. Kuczek, and J. R. Burgess, "Omega-3 Fatty Acids in Boys with Behavior, Learning, and Health Problems," *Physiology & Behavior* 59, no. 4–5 (April–May 1996): 915–20.

113 *Eating omega-3s has also been shown to alleviate the symptoms of depression:* M. P. Freeman et al., "Randomized Dose-Ranging Pilot Trial of Omega-3 Fatty Acids for Postpartum Depression," *Acta Psychiatrica Scandinavica* 113, no. 1 (January 2006): 31–35. See also C. L. Jensen, "Effects of N-3 Fatty Acids During Pregnancy and Lactation," *American Journal of Clinical Nutrition* 83, no. 6 Suppl. (June 2006): 1452S–57S.

113 *A 2008 study found fish oil:* S. Jazayeri et al., "Comparison of Therapeutic Effects of Omega-3 Fatty Acid Eicosapentaenoic Acid and Fluoxetine, Separately and in Combination, in Major Depressive Disorder," *Australian and New Zealand Journal of Psychiatry* 42, no. 3 (March 2008): 192–98.

114 *lycopene, helps maintain mood:* E. Gouranton et al., "Lycopene Inhibits Pro-inflammatory Cytokine and Chemokine Expression in Adipose Tissue," *Journal of Nutritional Biochemistry* 22, no. 7 (July 2011): 642–48.

114 *In a study of elderly nuns:* M. D. Gross and D. A. Snowdon, "Plasma Lycopene and Longevity: Findings from the Nun Study," *FASEB Journal* 15, No. 4 (March 7, 2001): A400. See also www.smart-publications.com/articles/lycopene-naringenin-and-chlorogenic-acid-the-health-benefits-of-tomato.

115 *it also contains a lot of citrulline:* A. M. Rimando and P. M. Perkins-Veazie, "Determination of Citrulline in Watermelon Rind," *Journal of Chromatography A* 1078, no. 1–2 (June 17, 2005): 196-200. See also www.sciencedaily.com/releases/2008/06/080630165707.htm.

115 *The red flesh of watermelon:* P. Perkins-Veazie, J. K. Collins, A. R. Davis, and W. Roberts, "Carotenoid Content of 50 Watermelon Cultivars," *Journal of Agricultural and Food Chemistry* 54, no. 7 (April 5, 2006): 2593–97. See also www.ars.usda.gov/is/AR/archive/jun02/lyco0602.htm.

115 *Studies show you can boost the levels:* P. Perkins-Veazie and J. K. Collins, "Carotenoid Changes of Intact Watermelons after Storage," *Journal of Agricultural and Food Chemistry* 54, no. 16 (August 9, 2006): 5868–74.

116 *capsaicin . . . cools our bodies and fights inflammation:* C. S. Kim et al., "Capsaicin Exhibits Anti-Inflammatory Property by Inhibiting Ikb-a Degradation in Lps-Stimulated Peritoneal Macrophages," *Cellular Signalling* 15, no. 3 (March 2003): 299–306.

116 *loaded with receptors for capsaicin:* E. Mezey et al., "Distribution of Mrna for Vanilloid Receptor Subtype 1 (Vr1), and Vr1-Like Immunoreactivity, in the Central Nervous System of the Rat and Human," *Proceedings of the National Academy of Sciences of the United States of America* 97, no. 7 (March 28, 2000): 3655–60.

116 *Capsaicin also destroys carcinogens:* Y. Avraham et al., "Capsaicin Affects Brain Function in a Model of Hepatic Encephalopathy Associated with Fulminant Hepatic Failure in Mice," *British Journal of Pharmacology* 158, no. 3 (October 2009): 896–906.

116 *capsaicin has been shown to protect the brain:* Y. Avraham et al., "Capsaicin Affects Brain Function in a Model of Hepatic Encephalopathy Associated with Fulminant Hepatic Failure in Mice," *British Journal of Pharmacology* 158, no. 3 (October 2009): 896–906.

120 *Uridine . . . stimulates the production of phosphotidylcholine*: R. J. Wurtman, M. Cansev, and I. H. Ulus, "Synapse Formation Is Enhanced by Oral Administration of Uridine and DHA, the Circulating Precursors of Brain Phosphatides," *Journal of Nutrition, Health & Aging* 13, no. 3 (March 2009): 189–97.

120 *A combination of uridine and omega-3s:* W.A. Carlezon et al., "Antidepressant-Like Effects of Uridine and Omega-3 Fatty Acids Are Potentiated by Combined Treatment in Rats," *Biological Psychiatry* 57, no. 4 (February 15, 2005): 343–50.

120 *Beets contain another phytonutrient family:* D. Strack, T. Vogt, and W. Schliemann, "Recent Advances in Betalain Research," *Phytochemistry* 62, no. 3 (February 2003): 247–69. See also C. H. Lee, M. Wettasinghe, B. W. Bolling, L. L. Ji, and K. L. Parkin, "Betalains, Phase Ii Enzyme-Inducing Components from Red Beetroot (Beta Vulgaris L.) Extracts," *Nutrition and Cancer* 53, no. 1 (2005): 91–103.

120 *These savory vegetables relax your blood vessels:* C. H. Lee, M. Wettasinghe, B. W. Bolling, L. L. Ji, and K. L. Parkin, "Betalains, Phase Ii Enzyme-Inducing Components from Red Beetroot (Beta Vulgaris L.) Extracts," *Nutrition and Cancer* 53, no. 1 (2005): 91–103. See also J. Koscielny et al., "The Antiatherosclerotic Effect of Allium Sativum," *Atherosclerosis* 144, no. 1 (May 1999): 237–49.

121 *it influences the uptake of tryptophan:* M. F. McCarty, "Enhancing Central and Peripheral Insulin Activity as a Strategy for the Treatment of Endogenous Depression—an Adjuvant Role for Chromium Picolinate?" *Medical Hypotheses* 43, no. 4 (October 1994): 247–52.

121 *Chromium supplementation is effective:* N. Iovieno, E. D. Dalton, M. Fava, and D. Mischoulon, "Second-Tier Natural Antidepressants: Review and Critique," *Journal of Affective Disorders* 130, no. 3 (May 2011): 343–57.

121 *Alliums lower blood sugar:* M. Thomson, K. K. Al-Qattan, T. Bordia, and M. Ali, "Including Garlic in the Diet May Help Lower Blood Glucose, Cholesterol, and Triglycerides," *Journal of Nutrition* 136, no. 3 Suppl. (March 2006): 800S–02S.

121 *allicin in garlic breaks up arterial plaques*: J. Koscielny et al., "The Antiatherosclerotic Effect of Allium Sativum," *Atherosclerosis* 144, no. 1 (May 1999): 237–49.

Select Notes for Top 100 Reasons
to Avoid Supplements

1: Burdock, G. A. "Safety Assessment of Castoreum Extract as a Food Ingredient." *International Journal of Toxicology* 26, no. 1 (2007): 51–5.

3: http://www.dunkindonuts.com/content/dunkindonuts/en/menu/donuts. html?DRP_FLAVOR=Glazed+Chocolate+Cake+Stick and http://food. oregonstate.edu/glossary/t/tertiarybutylhydroquinone.html

4: Julien, C., C. Tremblay, A. Phivilay, L. Berthiaume, V. Emond, P. Julien, and F. Calon. "High-Fat Diet Aggravates Amyloid-Beta and Tau Pathologies in the 3xtg-Ad Mouse Model." *Neurobiology of Aging* 31, no. 9 (2010): 1516–31.

6: Molteni, R., R. J. Barnard, Z. Ying, C. K. Roberts, and F. Gomez-Pinilla. "A High-Fat, Refined Sugar Diet Reduces Hippocampal Brain-Derived Neurotrophic Factor, Neuronal Plasticity, and Learning." *Neuroscience* 112, no. 4 (2002): 803–14.

7: Data compiled from http://www.whatsonmyfood.org/food.jsp?food=AC, based on the USDA Pesticide Data Program (http://www.ams.usda.gov/ AMSv1.0/getfile?dDocName=STELDEV3003674)

8: http://www.csmonitor.com/From-the-news-wires/2010/0716/Kellogg-cereal-recall-due-to-unusual-smells-in-box-liners

9: nutrition.mcdonalds.com/nutritionexchange/ingredientslist.pdf; and ntp. niehs.nih.gov/ntp/roc/twelfth/profiles/ButylatedHydroxyanisole.pdf

10: Interview with Smith Detection, World Wide Food Expo Chicago, IL October 28, 2009

16: http://www.nytimes.com/2010/03/12/business/12seed.html and http://www. cleveland.com/nation/index.ssf/2009/12/monsanto_uses_patent_law_to_ co.html

17: http://www.ucsusa.org/food_and_agriculture/science_and_impacts/ impacts_industrial_agriculture/they-eat-what-the-reality-of.html

19: http://health.msn.com/health-topics/cholesterol/fat-free-fat

20: http://www.vrg.org/nutshell/faqingredients.htm#cystine

21: http://www.epa.gov/oppsrrd1/REDs/factsheets/0003fact.pdf

22: Acero, S., A. I. Tabar, M. J. Alvarez, B. E. Garcia, J. M. Olaguibel, and I. Moneo. "Occupational Asthma and Food Allergy Due to Carmine." *Allergy* 53, no. 9 (1998): 897–901.

23: http://www.easylunchboxes.com/blog/whats-in-a-lunchable-a-healthier-homemade-alternative/

24: Costs for depression: Greenberg, P. E., R. C. Kessler, H. G. Birnbaum, S. A. Leong, S. W. Lowe, P. A. Berglund, and P. K. Corey-Lisle. "The Economic

Burden of Depression in the United States: How Did It Change between 1990 and 2000?" *Journal of Clinical Psychiatry* 64, no. 12 (2003): 1465–75; Alzheimer's: http://www.alz.org/downloads/Facts_Figures_2011.pdf; obesity: http://www.usatoday.com/yourlife/health/medical/2011-01-12-obesity-costs-300-bilion_N.htm; diabetes:174 billion http://www.diabetes.org/diabetes-basics/diabetes-statistics/

26: Wiles, N. J., K. Northstone, P. Emmett, and G. Lewis. "'Junk Food' Diet and Childhood Behavioural Problems: Results from the Alspac Cohort." *European Journal of Clinical Nutrition* 63, no. 4 (2009): 491–8.

27: Weese, J. S. "Methicillin-Resistant Staphylococcus Aureus in Animals." *ILAR J* 51, no. 3 (2010): 233–44.

28: Larsson S.C., Bergkvist L., Wolk A. "Processed meat consumption, dietary nitrosamines and stomach cancer risk in a cohort of Swedish women." *International Journal of Cancer.* 2006;119(4):915–9

29: http://www.associatedcontent.com/article/823337/the_dangers_of_the_additive_brominated.html; Horowitz, B. Z. "Bromism from Excessive Cola Consumption." *Journal of Toxicology-Clinical Toxicology* 35, no. 3 (1997): 315–20; Allain, P., S. Berre, N. Krari, P. Laine, N. Barbot, V. Rohmer, and J. C. Bigorgne. "Bromine and Thyroid Hormone Activity." *Journal of Clinical Pathology* 46, no. 5 (1993): 456–8.

30: Natah, S. S., K. R. Hussien, J. A. Tuominen, and V. A. Koivisto. "Metabolic Response to Lactitol and Xylitol in Healthy Men." *American Journal of Clinical Nutrition* 65, no. 4 (1997): 947–50.

31: Andres-Lacueva, C., B. Shukitt-Hale, R. L. Galli, O. Jauregui, R. M. Lamuela-Raventos, and J. A. Joseph. "Anthocyanins in Aged Blueberry-Fed Rats Are Found Centrally and May Enhance Memory." *Nutritional Neuroscience* 8, no. 2 (2005): 111–20; Galli, R. L., B. Shukitt-Hale, K. A. Youdim, and J. A. Joseph. "Fruit Polyphenolics and Brain Aging: Nutritional Interventions Targeting Age-Related Neuronal and Behavioral Deficits." *Annals of the New York Academy of Sciences* 959 (2002): 128–32; Schab, D. W., and N. H. Trinh. "Do Artificial Food Colors Promote Hyperactivity in Children with Hyperactive Syndromes? A Meta-Analysis of Double-Blind Placebo-Controlled Trials." *Journal of Developmental & Behavioral Pediatrics* 25, no. 6 (2004): 423–34.

32: http://www.shopwell.com/kraft-stove-top-stuffing-mix-chicken/doughs-mixes/p/4300028521; Amadasi, A., A. Mozzarelli, C. Meda, A. Maggi, and P. Cozzini. "Identification of Xenoestrogens in Food Additives by an Integrated in Silico and in Vitro Approach." *Chemical Research in Toxicology* 22, no. 1 (2009): 52–63.

35: Shapiro, A., W. Mu, C. Roncal, K. Y. Cheng, R. J. Johnson, and P. J. Scarpace. "Fructose-Induced Leptin Resistance Exacerbates Weight Gain in Response to Subsequent High-Fat Feeding." *American Journal of Physiology* 295, no. 5 (2008): R1370–5.

36, 39, 56, 59, 60: For a complete list of "Food defect action levels" see: http://

www.fda.gov/food/guidancecomplianceregulatoryinformation/guidancedocuments/sanitation/ucm056174.htm#intro

37: http://www.cnn.com/2010/HEALTH/10/16/veggie.recall/index.html

40: http://www.coffee-mate.com/Faqs.aspx; www.cspinet.org/nah/04_08/creamed.pdf

41: http://www.sciencedaily.com/releases/2010/06/100622112548.htm; Kohli, R., M. Kirby, S. A. Xanthakos, S. Softic, A. E. Feldstein, V. Saxena, P. H. Tang, L. Miles, M. V. Miles, W. F. Balistreri, S. C. Woods, and R. J. Seeley. "High-Fructose, Medium Chain Trans Fat Diet Induces Liver Fibrosis and Elevates Plasma Coenzyme Q9 in a Novel Murine Model of Obesity and Nonalcoholic Steatohepatitis." *Hepatology* 52, no. 3 (2010): 934–44.

42: http://monographs.iarc.fr/ENG/Monographs/PDFs/93-titaniumdioxide.pdf

43: White, L. R., H. Petrovitch, G. W. Ross, K. Masaki, J. Hardman, J. Nelson, D. Davis, and W. Markesbery. "Brain Aging and Midlife Tofu Consumption." *Journal of the American College of Nutrition* 19, no. 2 (2000): 242–55.

46: http://www.bloomberg.com/news/2011-05-18/amazon-deforestation-jumped-sixfold-on-expanded-soy-planting-brazil-says.html

47: http://www.nrdc.org/health/atrazine/

48: www.cspinet.org/new/pdf/food-dyes-rainbow-of-risks.pdf; http://www.scientificamerican.com/article.cfm?id=where-does-blue-food-dye

49: Micha, R., S. K. Wallace, and D. Mozaffarian. "Red and Processed Meat Consumption and Risk of Incident Coronary Heart Disease, Stroke, and Diabetes Mellitus: A Systematic Review and Meta-Analysis." *Circulation* 121, no. 21 (2010): 2271–83.

50: Risérus, U., L. Berglund, and B. Vessby. "Conjugated Linoleic Acid (Cla) Reduced Abdominal Adipose Tissue in Obese Middle-Aged Men with Signs of the Metabolic Syndrome: A Randomised Controlled Trial." *International Journal of Obesity and Related Metabolic Disorders* 25, no. 8 (2001): 1129–35.

51: http://www.youtube.com/watch?v=eSIcPiIAeIE

52: http://www2.kelloggs.com/ProductDetail.aspx?id=2538

53: http://www.time.com/time/health/article/0,8599,1711763,00.html; Davidson, T. L., and S. E. Swithers. "A Pavlovian Approach to the Problem of Obesity." *International Journal of Obesity and Related Metabolic Disorders* 28, no. 7 (2004): 933–5.

54: http://eur-lex.europa.eu/LexUriServ/LexUriServ.do?uri=OJ:L:2004:007:0045:0046:EN:PDF

55: Chavarro, J. E., T. L. Toth, S. M. Sadio, and R. Hauser. "Soy Food and Isoflavone Intake in Relation to Semen Quality Parameters among Men from an Infertility Clinic." *Human Reproduction* 23, no. 11 (2008): 2584–90; http://www.independent.co.uk/life-style/health-and-families/health-news/soya-products-linked-to-low-sperm-count-876053.html

57: http://www.thesmokinggun.com/documents/crime/mcnuggets-rage

58: http://www.cbsnews.com/stories/2011/04/05/health/main20050766.shtml

63: Smit, L. A., A. Baylin, and H. Campos. "Conjugated Linoleic Acid in Adipose Tissue and Risk of Myocardial Infarction." *American Journal of Clinical Nutrition* 92, no. 1 (2010): 34–40.

67: http://www.washingtonpost.com/wp-dyn/content/article/2008/12/29/AR2008122901204.html

68: http://www.sciencedaily.com/releases/2009/01/090127083638.htm

69: http://news.bbc.co.uk/2/hi/health/4115506.stm

70: http://www.cdc.gov/ncidod/dbmd/diseaseinfo/salmonellosis_2007/outbreak_notice.htm

71: Li, S., J. H. Zhao, J. Luan, R. N. Luben, S. A. Rodwell, K. T. Khaw, K. K. Ong, N. J. Wareham, and R. J. Loos. "Cumulative Effects and Predictive Value of Common Obesity-Susceptibility Variants Identified by Genome-Wide Association Studies." *American Journal of Clinical Nutrition* 91, no. 1 (2010): 184–90.

72: http://www.foodandwaterwatch.org/reports/suspicious-shrimp/

73: http://abcnews.go.com/GMA/OnCall/story?id=3565670&page=1

76: http://www.fsis.usda.gov/News_&_Events/Recall_060_2011_Release/index.asp

79: http://www.bbc.co.uk/worldservice/specials/1616_fastfood/page6.shtml

81: Nestle, Marion. *Food Politics : How the Food Industry Influences Nutrition and Health*, California Studies in Food and Culture. Berkeley: University of California Press, 2002 (68).

83: http://civileats.com/2010/10/01/rbgh-free-claim-ruled-ok-with-no-caveats/

85: http://grassfedcooking.com/2009/pastured-pork-and-foodborne-pathogens/

86: http://www.nytimes.com/2011/02/11/business/11tyson.html

87: http://www.fda.gov/Safety/Recalls/ucm241359.htm

89: MacLusky, N. J., T. Hajszan, and C. Leranth. "The Environmental Estrogen Bisphenol a Inhibits Estradiol-Induced Hippocampal Synaptogenesis." *Environ Health Perspect* 113, no. 6 (2005): 675-9.

Hajszan, T., and C. Leranth. "Bisphenol a Interferes with Synaptic Remodeling." *Frontiers in Neuroendocrinology* 31, no. 4 (2010): 519–30.

90: McCann, D., A. Barrett, A. Cooper, D. Crumpler, L. Dalen, K. Grimshaw, E. Kitchin, K. Lok, L. Porteous, E. Prince, E. Sonuga-Barke, J. O. Warner, and J. Stevenson. "Food Additives and Hyperactive Behaviour in 3-Year-Old and 8/9-Year-Old Children in the Community: A Randomised, Double-Blinded, Placebo-Controlled Trial." *Lancet* 370, no. 9598 (2007): 1560–7.

92: http://news.ncsu.edu/releases/014mkschalantibiotic; Ahmad, A., A. Ghosh, C. Schal, and L. Zurek. "Insects in Confined Swine Operations Carry a Large Antibiotic Resistant and Potentially Virulent Enterococcal Community." *BMC Microbiology* 11, no. 1 (2011): 23.

95: http://www.huffingtonpost.com/2011/01/25/taco-bell-beef-lawsuit_n_813185.html

97: http://foodsafety.einnews.com/article/1634-harmful-chemicals-showing-up-in-fast-food-wrappers;

D'eon, J. C., and S. A. Mabury. "Exploring Indirect Sources of Human Exposure to Perfluoroalkyl Carboxylates (Pfcas): Evaluating Uptake, Elimination, and Biotransformation of Polyfluoroalkyl Phosphate Esters (Paps) in the Rat." *Environmental Health Perspectives* 119, no. 3 (2011): 344–50.

100: Ozanne, S. E., and C. N. Hales. "The Long-Term Consequences of Intra-Uterine Protein Malnutrition for Glucose Metabolism." *Proc Nutr Soc* 58, no. 3 (1999): 615–9.

Selected References

Abdolmaleky HM, Smith CL, Zhou JR, Thiagalingam S. Epigenetic alterations of the dopaminergic system in major psychiatric disorders. *Methods Mol Biol.* 2008;448:187–212.

Acero, S., A. I. Tabar, M. J. Alvarez, B. E. Garcia, J. M. Olaguibel, and I. Moneo. "Occupational Asthma and Food Allergy Due to Carmine." Allergy 53, no. 9 (1998): 897–901.

Ahmad, A., A. Ghosh, C. Schal, and L. Zurek. "Insects in Confined Swine Operations Carry a Large Antibiotic Resistant and Potentially Virulent Enterococcal Community." *BMC Microbiol* 11, no. 1 (2011): 23.

Akbaraly TN, Brunner EJ, Ferrie JE, Marmot MG, Kivimaki M, Singh-Manoux A. Dietary pattern and depressive symptoms in middle age. *Br J Psychiatry.* 2009 Nov;195(5):408–13.

Allain, P., S. Berre, N. Krari, P. Laine, N. Barbot, V. Rohmer, and J. C. Bigorgne. "Bromine and Thyroid Hormone Activity." *J Clin Pathol* 46, no. 5 (1993): 456–8.

Almoosawi S, Fyfe L, Ho C, Al-Dujaili E. The effect of polyphenol-rich dark chocolate on fasting capillary whole blood glucose, total cholesterol, blood pressure and glucocorticoids in healthy overweight and obese subjects. *Br J Nutr.* 2010 Mar;103(6):842–50.

Amadasi, A., A. Mozzarelli, C. Meda, A. Maggi, and P. Cozzini. "Identification of Xenoestrogens in Food Additives by an Integrated in Silico and in Vitro Approach." *Chem Res Toxicol* 22, no. 1 (2009): 52–63.

Amagase H, Petesch BL, Matsuura H, Kasuga S, Itakura Y. Intake of garlic and its bioactive components. *J Nutr.* 2001 Mar;131(3s):955S–62S.

Amminger GP, Schäfer MR, Papageorgiou K, Klier CM, Cotton SM, Harrigan SM, Mackinnon A, McGorry PD, Berger GE. Long-chain omega-3 fatty acids for indicated prevention of psychotic disorders: a randomized, placebo-controlled trial. *Arch Gen Psychiatry.* 2010 Feb;67(2):146–54.

Anderson JW, Baird P, Davis RH Jr, Ferreri S, Knudtson M, Koraym A, Waters V, Williams CL. Health benefits of dietary fiber. *Nutr Rev.* 2009 Apr;67(4):188–205.

Andres-Lacueva, C., B. Shukitt-Hale, R. L. Galli, O. Jauregui, R. M. Lamuela-

Raventos, and J. A. Joseph. "Anthocyanins in Aged Blueberry-Fed Rats Are Found Centrally and May Enhance Memory." *Nutr Neurosci* 8, no. 2 (2005): 111–20.

Angela Liou Y, Innis SM. Dietary linoleic acid has no effect on arachidonic acid, but increases n-6 eicosadienoic acid, and lowers dihomo-gamma-linolenic and eicosapentaenoic acid in plasma of adult men. *Prostaglandins Leukot Essent Fatty Acids.* 2009 Apr;80(4):201–6.

Arterburn LM, Hall EB, Oken H. Distribution, interconversion, and dose response of n-3 fatty acids in humans. *Am J Clin Nutr.* 2006 Jun;83(6 Suppl):1467S–76S.

Arterburn LM, Hall EB, Oken H. Distribution, interconversion, and dose response of n-3 fatty acids in humans. *Am J Clin Nutr.* 2006 Jun;83(6 Suppl):1467S–76S.

Banni S, Petroni A, Blasevich M, Carta G, Cordeddu L, Murru E, Melis MP, Mahon A, Belury MA. Conjugated linoleic acids (CLA) as precursors of a distinct family of PUFA. *Lipids.* 2004 Nov;39(11):1143–46.

Bantle JP. Dietary fructose and metabolic syndrome and diabetes. *J Nutr.* 2009 Jun;139(6):1263S–68S.

Batterham RL, Heffron H, Kapoor S, Chivers J, Chandarana K, Herzog H, Le Roux CW, Thomas EL, Bell JD, Withers DJ. Critical role for peptide YY in protein-mediated satiation and body-weight regulation. *Cell Metabolism.* 2006;4(3):223–33.

Berry SE. Triacylglycerol structure and interesterification of palmitic and stearic acid-rich fats: an overview and implications for cardiovascular disease. *Nutr Res Rev.* 2009 Jun;22(1):3–17.

Bes-Rastrollo M, Wedick NM, Martinez-Gonzalez MA, Li TY, Sampson L, Hu FB.Prospective study of nut consumption, long-term weight change, and obesity risk in women. *Am J Clin Nutr.* 2009 Jun;89(6):1913–19.

Bjelland I, Tell GS, Vollset SE, Konstantinova S, Ueland PM. Choline in anxiety and depression: the Hordaland Health Study. *Am J Clin Nutr.* 2009 Oct;90(4):1056–60.

Bocarsly ME, Powell ES, Avena NM, Hoebel BG. High-fructose corn syrup causes characteristics of obesity in rats: Increased body weight, body fat and triglyceride levels. *Pharmacol Biochem Behav.* 2010 Feb 26.

Bodnar LM et al. High prevalence of vitamin D insufficiency in black and white pregnant women residing in the northern United States and their neonates. *J. Nutr.* 2007 Feb;137(2):447–52.

Bonnet E, Touyarot K, Alfos S, Pallet V, Higueret P, et al. Retinoic acid restores adult hippocampal neurogenesis and reverses spatial memory deficit in vitamin A deprived rats. *PLoS One.* 2008;3(10):e3487. doi:10.1371/journal.pone.0003487

Boots AW, Haenen GR, Bast A. Health effects of quercetin: from antioxidant to nutraceutical. *Eur J Pharmacol.* 2008 May 13;585(2–3):325–37.

Bradford GS, Taylor CT. Omeprazole and vitamin B12 deficiency. *Ann Pharmacother.* 1999 May;33(5):641–43.

Brenna JT, Salem N Jr, Sinclair AJ, Cunnane SC. alpha-Linolenic acid supplementation and conversion to n-3 long-chain polyunsaturated fatty acids in humans. *Prostaglandins Leukot Essent Fatty Acids.* 2009 Feb–Mar;80(2–3):85–91.

Brunoni AR, Lopes M, Fregni F. A systematic review and meta-analysis of clinical studies on major depression and BDNF levels: implications for the role of neuroplasticity in depression. *Int J Neuropsychopharmacol.* 2008 Dec;11(8):1169–80. doi:10.1017/S1461145708009309.

Camire ME, Kubow S, Donnelly DJ. Potatoes and human health. *Crit Rev Food Sci Nutr.* 2009 Nov;49(10):823–40.

Cannell JJ et al. Epidemic influenza and vitamin *D. Epidemiol Infect.* 2006 Dec;134(6):1129-40.

Carlezon WA Jr, Mague SD, Parow AM, Stoll AL, Cohen BM, Renshaw PF. Antidepressant-like effects of uridine and omega-3 fatty acids are potentiated by combined treatment in rats. *Biol Psychiatry,* 2005 Feb;57(4):343–50.

Chavarro, J. E., T. L. Toth, S. M. Sadio, and R. Hauser. "Soy Food and Isoflavone Intake in Relation to Semen Quality Parameters among Men from an Infertility Clinic." *Hum Reprod* 23, no. 11 (2008): 2584–90.

Cheng S. Adiposity, cardiometabolic risk, and vitamin D status: the Framingham Heart Study. *Diabetes.* 2010 Jan;59(1):242–48.

Cohen PG. Obesity in men: the hypogonadal-estrogen receptor relationship and its effect on glucose homeostasis. *Med Hypotheses.* 2008;70(2):358–60.

Conklin SM, Gianaros PJ, Brown SM, Yao JK, Hariri AR, Manuck SB, Muldoon MF. Long-chain omega-3 fatty acid intake is associated positively with corticolimbic gray matter volume in healthy adults. *Neurosci Lett.* 2007 Jun 29;421(3):209–12.

Cordain L, Lindeberg S, Hurtado M, Hill K, Eaton SB, Brand-Miller J. Acne vulgaris: a disease of western civilization. *Arch Dermatol.* 2002;138:1584–90.

Corniola RS, Tassabehji NM, Hare J, Sharma G, Levenson CW. Zinc deficiency impairs neuronal precursor cell proliferation and induces apoptosis via p53-mediated mechanisms. *Brain Res.* 2008 Oct 27;1237:52–61.

Costa J, Lunet N, Santos C, Santos J, Vaz-Carneiro A. Caffeine exposure and the risk of Parkinson's disease: a systematic review and meta-analysis of observational studies. *J Alzheimers Dis.* 2010;20 Suppl 1:S221–38.

Craig SA. Betaine in human nutrition. *Am J Clin Nutr.* 2004 Sep;80(3):539–49.

D'eon, J. C., and S. A. Mabury. "Exploring Indirect Sources of Human Exposure to Perfluoroalkyl Carboxylates (Pfcas): Evaluating Uptake, Elimination, and Biotransformation of Polyfluoroalkyl Phosphate Esters (Paps) in the Rat." *Environ Health Perspect* 119, no. 3 (2011): 344–50.

Davidson, T. L., and S. E. Swithers. "A Pavlovian Approach to the Problem of Obesity." *Int J Obes Relat Metab Disord* 28, no. 7 (2004): 933–5.

de la Monte SM, Wands JR. Alzheimer's disease is type 3 diabetes—evidence reviewed. *J Diabetes Sci Technol.* 2008 Nov;2(6):1101–13.

Dimopoulos N, Piperi C, Salonicioti A, Psarra V, Mitsonis C, Liappas I, Lea RW, Kalofoutis A. Characterization of the lipid profile in dementia and depression in the elderly. *J Geriatr Psychiatry Neurol.* 2007 Sep;20(3):138–44.

Ellis, Carleton. *The Hydrogenation of Oils: Catalyzers and Catalysis and the Generation of Hydrogen and Oxygen.* Second edition 1919. D. Van Nordstrand Company. New York.

Ervin RB. Prevalence of metabolic syndrome among adults 20 years of age and over, by sex, age, race and ethnicity, and body mass index: United States 2003–2006. National Health Statistics Reports. 2009;13:1–8. Available at http://www.cdc.gov/nchs/nhanes/new_nhanes.htm.

Eskelinen MH, Kivipelto M. Caffeine as a protective factor in dementia and Alzheimer's disease. *J Alzheimers Dis.* 2010;20 Suppl 1:S167–74.

Fahey JW, Haristoy X, Dolan PM, Kensler TW, Scholtus I, Stephenson KK, Talalay P, Lozniewski A. Sulforaphane inhibits extracellular, intracellular, and antibiotic-resistant strains of Helicobacter pylori and prevents benzo[a]pyrene-induced stomach tumors. *Proc Natl Acad Sci USA.* 2002 May 28;99(11):7610–15.

Fisher ND, Sorond FA, Hollenberg NK. Cocoa flavanols and brain perfusion. *J Cardiovasc Pharmacol.* 2006;47 Suppl 2:S210–14.

Fortuna JL. Sweet preference, sugar addiction and the familial history of alcohol dependence: shared neural pathways and genes. *J Psychoactive Drugs.* 2010 Jun;42(2):147–51.

Galeone C, Pelucchi C, Levi F, Negri E, Franceschi S, Talamini R, Giacosa A, La Vecchia C. Onion and garlic use and human cancer. *Am J Clin Nutr.* 2006 Nov;84(5):1027–32.

Galli, R. L., B. Shukitt-Hale, K. A. Youdim, and J. A. Joseph. "Fruit Polyphenolics and Brain Aging: Nutritional Interventions Targeting Age-Related Neuronal and Behavioral Deficits." *Ann N Y Acad Sci* 959 (2002): 128–32.

Gaullier JM, Halse J, Høye K, Kristiansen K, Fagertun H, Vik H, Gudmundsen O. Supplementation with conjugated linoleic acid for 24 months is well tolerated by and reduces body fat mass in healthy, overweight humans. *J Nutr.* 2005 Apr;135(4):778–84.

Gouranton E, Thabuis C, Riollet C, Malezet-Desmoulins C, El Yazidi C, Amiot MJ, Borel P, Landrier JF. Lycopene inhibits proinflammatory cytokine and chemokine expression in adipose tissue. *J Nutr Biochem.* 2010 Oct 15.

Gow RV, Matsudaira T, Taylor E, Rubia K, Crawford M, Ghebremeskel K, Ibrahimovic A, Vallée-Tourangeau F, Williams LM, Sumich A. Total red blood cell concentrations of omega-3 fatty acids are associated with emotion-elicited neural activity in adolescent boys with attention-deficit hyperactivity disorder. *Prostaglandins Leukot Essent Fatty Acids.* 2009 Feb-Mar;80(2–3):151–56.

Gow RV, Matsudaira T, Taylor E, Rubia K, Crawford M, Ghebremeskel K, Ibrahimovic A, Vallée-Tourangeau F, Williams LM, Sumich A. Total red blood cell concentrations of omega-3 fatty acids are associated with emotion-elicited neural activity in adolescent boys with attention-deficit hyperactivity disorder. *Prostaglandins Leukot Essent Fatty Acids.* 2009 Feb-Mar;80(2–3):151–56.

Greenberg, P. E., R. C. Kessler, H. G. Birnbaum, S. A. Leong, S. W. Lowe, P. A. Berglund, and P. K. Corey-Lisle. "The Economic Burden of Depression in the United States: How Did It Change between 1990 and 2000?" *J Clin Psychiatry* 64, no. 12 (2003): 1465–75.

Gunstad J et al. Improved memory function 12 weeks after bariatric surgery. *Surg Obes Relat Dis.* 2010 Oct 4. doi:10.1016/j.soard.2010.09.015.

Ha SO, Yoo HJ, Park SY, Hong HS, Kim DS, Cho HJ. Capsaicin effects on brain-derived neurotrophic factor in rat dorsal root ganglia and spinal cord. *Brain Res Mol Brain Res.* 2000 Sep 30;81(1–2):181–86.

Hadjipavlou-Litina D, Garnelis T, Athanassopoulos CM, Papaioannou D. Kukoamine A analogs with lipoxygenase inhibitory activity. *J Enzyme Inhib Med Chem.* 2009 Oct;24(5):1188–93.

Hajszan, T., and C. Leranth. "Bisphenol a Interferes with Synaptic Remodeling." *Front Neuroendocrinol* 31, no. 4 (2010): 519–30.

Halvorsen BL, Carlsen MH, Phillips KM, Bøhn SK, Holte K, Jacobs DR Jr, Blomhoff R. Content of redox-active compounds (ie, antioxidants) in foods consumed in the United States. *Am J Clin Nutr.* 2006 Jul;84(1):95–135.

Henderson VW, Guthrie JR, Dennerstein L. Serum lipids and memory in a population based cohort of middle age women. *J Neurol Neurosurg Psychiatry.* 2003 Nov;74(11):1530–35.

Herraiz T, Chaparro C. Human monoamine oxidase enzyme inhibition by coffee and beta-carbolines norharman and harman isolated from coffee. *Life Sci.* 2006 Jan 18;78(8):795–802.

Holt S, Brand J, Soveny C, Hansky J. Relationship of satiety to postprandial glycaemic, insulin and cholecystokinin responses. *Appetite.* 1992 Apr;18(2):129–41.

Horlick L, Katz LN. The relationship of atheromatosis development in the chicken to the amount of cholesterol added to the diet. *Am Heart J.* 1949 Sep;38(3):336–49.

Horowitz, B. Z. "Bromism from Excessive Cola Consumption." *J Toxicol Clin Toxicol* 35, no. 3 (1997): 315–20.

Hu FB, Stampfer MJ, Rimm EB, Manson JE, Ascherio A, Colditz GA, Rosner BA, Spiegelman D, Speizer FE, Sacks FM, Hennekens CH, Willett WC. A prospective study of egg consumption and risk of cardiovascular disease in men and women. *JAMA.* 1999 Apr 21;281(15):1387–94.

Hudson C, Hudson S, MacKenzie J. Protein-source tryptophan as an efficacious treatment for social anxiety disorder: a pilot study. *Can J Physiol Pharmacol.* 2007 Sep;85(9):928–32.

Huxley R, Lee CM, Barzi F, Timmermeister L, Czernichow S, Perkovic V, Grobbee DE, Batty D, Woodward M. Coffee, decaffeinated coffee, and tea consumption in relation to incident type 2 diabetes mellitus: a systematic review with meta-analysis. *Arch Intern Med.* 2009 Dec 14;169(22):2053–63.

Ige SF, Akhigbe RE, Akinsanya AO. The role of hyperglycemia in skin wrinkle formation: Mediation of advanced glycation end-products. *Research Journal of Medical Sciences.* 2010;4(5):324–29.

Jacka FN, Kremer PJ, Leslie ER, Berk M, Patton GC, Toumbourou JW, Williams JW. Associations between diet quality and depressed mood in adolescents: results from the Australian Healthy Neighbourhoods Study. *Aust N Z J Psychiatry.* 2010 May;44(5):435–42.

Jacka FN, Pasco JA, Mykletun A, Williams LJ, Hodge AM, O'Reilly SL, Nicholson GC, Kotowicz MA, Berk M. Association of Western and traditional diets with depression and anxiety in women. *Am J Psychiatry.* 2010 Mar;167(3):305–11. doi:10.1176/ajp.2009.09060881.

Jagtap S, Meganathan K, Wagh V, Winkler J, Hescheler J, Sachinidis A.Chemoprotective mechanism of the natural compounds, epigallocatechin-3-O-gallate, quercetin and curcumin against cancer and cardiovascular diseases. *Curr Med Chem.* 2009;16(12):1451–62.

Jones PJ. Dietary cholesterol and the risk of cardiovascular disease in patients: a review of the Harvard Egg Study and other data. *Int J Clin Pract Suppl.* 2009 Oct;(163):1–8, 28–36.

Joo NE, Park CS. Inhibition of excitotoxicity in cultured rat cortical neurons by a mixture of conjugated linoleic acid isomers. *Pharmacol Res.* 2003 Apr;47(4):305–10.

Joseph JA, Shukitt-Hale B, Willis LM. Grape juice, berries, and walnuts affect brain aging and behavior. *J Nutr.* 2009 Sep;139(9):1813S–17S.

Julien, C., C. Tremblay, A. Phivilay, L. Berthiaume, V. Emond, P. Julien, and F. Calon. "High-Fat Diet Aggravates Amyloid-Beta and Tau Pathologies in the 3xtg-Ad Mouse Model." *Neurobiol Aging* 31, no. 9 (2010): 1516–31.

Kamata Y, Shiraga H, Tai A, Kawamoto Y, Gohda E. Induction of neurite outgrowth in PC12 cells by the medium-chain fatty acid octanoic acid. *Neuroscience.* 2007 May 25;146(3):1073–81.

Kawachi I, Willett WC, Colditz GA, Stampfer MJ, Speizer FE. A prospective study of coffee drinking and suicide in women. *Arch Intern Med.* 1996 Mar 11;156(5):521–25.

Kawai Y, Nishikawa T, Shiba Y, Saito S, Murota K, Shibata N, Kobayashi M, Kanayama M, Uchida K, Terao J. Macrophage as a target of quercetin glucuronides in human atherosclerotic arteries: implication in the anti-atherosclerotic mechanism of dietary flavonoids. *J Biol Chem.* 2008 Apr 4;283(14):9424–34.

Kelly JH Jr, Sabaté J. Nuts and coronary heart disease: an epidemiological perspective. *Br J Nutr.* 2006 Nov;96 Suppl 2:S61–67.

Kempf K, Herder C, Erlund I, Kolb H, Martin S, Carstensen M, Koenig W, Sundvall J, Bidel S, Kuha S, Jaakko T. Effects of coffee consumption on subclinical inflammation and other risk factors for type 2 diabetes: a clinical trial. *Am J Clin Nutr.* 2010 Apr;91(4):950–57.

Kessler RC, Berglund P, Demler O, et al. Lifetime prevalence and age-of-onset distributions of DSM-IV disorders in the National Comorbidity Survey Replication. *Arch Gen Psychiatry.* 2005;62:593–602.

Kohli, R., M. Kirby, S. A. Xanthakos, S. Softic, A. E. Feldstein, V. Saxena, P. H. Tang, L. Miles, M. V. Miles, W. F. Balistreri, S. C. Woods, and R. J. Seeley. "High-Fructose, Medium Chain Trans Fat Diet Induces Liver Fibrosis and Elevates Plasma Coenzyme Q9 in a Novel Murine Model of Obesity and Nonalcoholic Steatohepatitis." *Hepatology* 52, no. 3 (2010): 934–44.

Koscielny J, Klüssendorf D, Latza R, Schmitt R, Radtke H, Siegel G, Kiesewetter H. The antiatherosclerotic effect of Allium sativum. *Atherosclerosis.* 1999 May;144(1):237–49.

Krishnan K. More optimal forms of vitamin. *J Am Diet Assoc.* 2005 Feb;105(2): 204-5.

Kwon YI, Apostolidis E, Kim YC, Shetty K. Health benefits of traditional corn, beans, and pumpkin: in vitro studies for hyperglycemia and hypertension management. *J Med Food.* 2007 Jun;10(2):266–75.

Levenson CW, Morris. Zinc and Neurogenesis: Making new neurons from development to adulthood. *Adv Nutr.* 2011;2:96–100. doi:10.3945/an.110.000174.

Li, S., J. H. Zhao, J. Luan, R. N. Luben, S. A. Rodwell, K. T. Khaw, K. K. Ong, N. J. Wareham, and R. J. Loos. "Cumulative Effects and Predictive Value of Common Obesity-Susceptibility Variants Identified by Genome-Wide Association Studies." *Am J Clin Nutr* 91, no. 1 (2010): 184–90.

Liou YA, King DJ, Zibrik D, Innis SM. Decreasing linoleic acid with constant alpha-linolenic acid in dietary fats increases (n-3) eicosapentaenoic acid in plasma phospholipids in healthy men. *J Nutr.* 2007 Apr;137(4):945–52.

Lukiw WJ, Cui JG, Marcheselli VL, Bodker M, Botkjaer A, Gotlinger K, Serhan CN, Bazan NG. A role for docosahexaenoic acid-derived neuroprotectin D1 in neural cell survival and Alzheimer disease. *J Clin Invest.* 2005 Oct;115(10):2774–83.

Lukiw WJ, Cui JG, Marcheselli VL, Bodker M, Botkjaer A, Gotlinger K, Serhan CN, Bazan NG. A role for docosahexaenoic acid-derived neuroprotectin D1 in neural cell survival and Alzheimer disease. *J Clin Invest.* 2005 Oct;115(10):2774–83.

Lustman PJ, Anderson RJ, Freedland KE, de Groot M, Carney RM, Clouse RE. Depression and poor glycemic control: a meta-analytic review of the literature. *Diabetes Care.* 2000 Jul;23(7):934–42.

Lustman PJ, Anderson RJ, Freedland KE, de Groot M, Carney RM, Clouse RE.

Depression and poor glycemic control: a meta-analytic review of the literature. *Diabetes Care.* 2000 Jul;23(7):934–42.

Lütjohann D. Brain cholesterol and suicidal behaviour. *Int J Neuropsychopharmacol.* 2007 Apr;10(2):153–57.

Maes M et al. Lower serum vitamin E concentrations in major depression. Another marker of lowered antioxidant defenses in that illness. *J Affect Disord.* 2000 Jun;58(3):241–46.

Maguire LS, O'Sullivan SM, Galvin K, O'Connor TP, O'Brien NM. Fatty acid profile, tocopherol, squalene and phytosterol content of walnuts, almonds, peanuts, hazelnuts and the macadamia nut. *Int J Food Sci Nutr.* 2004 May;55(3):171–78.

Manderbacka K, Sund R, Koski S, Keskimäki I, Elovainio M. Diabetes and depression? Secular trends in the use of antidepressants among persons with diabetes in Finland in 1997–2007. *Pharmacoepidemiol Drug Saf.* 2011 Apr;20(4):338–43. doi:10.1002/pds.2072.

Mann N. Dietary lean red meat and human evolution. *Eur J Nutr.* 2000 Apr;39(2):71–79.

Mann NJ, Ponnampalam EN, Yep Y, Sinclair AJ. Feeding regimes affect fatty acid composition in Australian beef cattle. *Asia Pac J Clin Nutr.* 2003;12 Suppl:S38.

Maras JE et al. Intake of alpha-tocopherol is limited among US adults. *J Am Diet Assoc.* 2004 Apr;104(4):567–75.

McCann, D., A. Barrett, A. Cooper, D. Crumpler, L. Dalen, K. Grimshaw, E. Kitchin, K. Lok, L. Porteous, E. Prince, E. Sonuga-Barke, J. O. Warner, and J. Stevenson. "Food Additives and Hyperactive Behaviour in 3-Year-Old and 8/9-Year-Old Children in the Community: A Randomised, Double-Blinded, Placebo-Controlled Trial." *Lancet* 370, no. 9598 (2007): 1560–7.

McIntyre RS, Kenna HA, Nguyen HT, Law CW, Sultan F, Woldeyohannes HO, Adams AK, Cheng JS, Lourenco M, Kennedy SH, Rasgon NL. Brain volume abnormalities and neurocognitive deficits in diabetes mellitus: points of pathophysiological commonality with mood disorders? *Adv Ther.* 2010 Feb;27(2):63–8Micha, R., S. K. Wallace, and D. Mozaffarian. "Red and Processed Meat Consumption and Risk of Incident Coronary Heart Disease, Stroke, and Diabetes Mellitus: A Systematic Review and Meta-Analysis." *Circulation* 121, no. 21 (2010): 2271–83.

Miller AH, Maletic V, Raison CL. Inflammation and its discontents: the role of cytokines in the pathophysiology of major depression. *Biol Psychiatry.* 2009 May 1;65(9):732–41.

Molteni, R., R. J. Barnard, Z. Ying, C. K. Roberts, and F. Gomez-Pinilla. "A High-Fat, Refined Sugar Diet Reduces Hippocampal Brain-Derived Neurotrophic Factor, Neuronal Plasticity, and Learning." *Neuroscience* 112, no. 4 (2002): 803–14.

Morris MC et al. Relation of the tocopherol forms to incident Alzheimer disease and to cognitive change. *Am J Clin Nutr.* 2005 Feb;81(2):508–14.

Morris MC, Evans DA, Tangney CC, Bienias JL, Wilson RS. Associations of vegetable and fruit consumption with age-related cognitive change. *Neurology.* 2006 Oct 24;67(8):1370–76.

Mozaffarian D, Clarke R. Quantitative effects on cardiovascular risk factors and coronary heart disease risk of replacing partially hydrogenated vegetable oils with other fats and oils. *Eur J Clin Nutr.* 2009 May;63 Suppl 2:S22–33.

Muldoon MF, Ryan CM, Sheu L, Yao JK, Conklin SM, Manuck SB. Serum phospholipid docosahexaenonic acid is associated with cognitive functioning during middle adulthood. *J Nutr.* 2010 Apr;140(4):848–53.

Natah, S. S., K. R. Hussien, J. A. Tuominen, and V. A. Koivisto. "Metabolic Response to Lactitol and Xylitol in Healthy Men." *Am J Clin Nutr* 65, no. 4 (1997): 947–50.

Nestle, Marion. *Food Politics : How the Food Industry Influences Nutrition and Health*, California Studies in Food and Culture. Berkeley: University of California Press, 2002.

Numakawa T, Suzuki S, Kumamaru E, Adachi N, Richards M, Kunugi H. BDNF function and intracellular signaling in neurons. *Histol Histopathol.* 2010 Feb;25(2):23758.

Oomah BD, Corbé A, Balasubramanian P. Antioxidant and anti-inflammatory activities of bean (Phaseolus vulgaris L.) hulls. *J Agric Food Chem.* 2010 Jul 28;58(14):8225–30.

Oyagbemi AA, Saba AB, Azeez OI. Capsaicin: a novel chemopreventive molecule and its underlying molecular mechanisms of action. *Indian J Cancer.* 2010 Jan-Mar;47(1):53–58.

Ozanne, S. E., and C. N. Hales. "The Long-Term Consequences of Intra-Uterine Protein Malnutrition for Glucose Metabolism." *Proc Nutr Soc* 58, no. 3 (1999): 615–9.

Papakostas GI et al. Cholesterol in mood and anxiety disorders: review of the literature and new hypotheses. *Eur Neuropsychopharmacol.* 2004 Mar;14(2):135–42.

Pelsser LM, Frankena K, Toorman J, Savelkoul HF, Dubois AE, Pereira RR, Haagen TA, Rommelse NN, Buitelaar JK. Effects of a restricted elimination diet on the behaviour of children with attention-deficit hyperactivity disorder (INCA study): a randomised controlled trial. *Lancet.* 2011 Feb 5;377(9764):494–503. doi:10.1016/S0140-6736(10)62227-1.

Pennington NL, Baker CW. Sugar Beets and Napoleon: Sugar, a user's guide to sucrose. http://www.archive.org/stream/sugarbeetinameri00harrrich#page/n7/mode/2up (The 1919 book *The Sugar-Beet In America* re movement of beet from Europe to USA).

Pereira MA, Parker ED, Folsom AR. Coffee consumption and risk of type 2 diabetes mellitus: an 11-year prospective study of 28 812 postmenopausal women. *Arch Intern Med.* 2006 Jun 26;166(12):1311–16.

Phillips KM, Carlsen MH, Blomhoff R. Total antioxidant content of alternatives to refined sugar. *J Am Diet Assoc.* 2009 Jan;109(1):64–71.

Pifferi F, Jouin M, Alessandri JM, Haedke U, Roux F, Perrière N, Denis I, Lavialle M, Guesnet P. n-3 Fatty acids modulate brain glucose transport in endothelial cells of the blood-brain barrier. *Prostaglandins Leukot Essent Fatty Acids.* 2007 Nov–Dec;77(5–6):279–86.

Ponte PI, Prates JA, Crespo JP, Crespo DG, Mourão JL, Alves SP, Bessa RJ, Chaveiro-Soares MA, Gama LT, Ferreira LM, Fontes CM. Restricting the intake of a cereal-based feed in free-range-pastured poultry: effects on performance and meat quality. *Poult Sci.* 2008 Oct;87(10):2032–42.

Risérus, U., L. Berglund, and B. Vessby. "Conjugated Linoleic Acid (Cla) Reduced Abdominal Adipose Tissue in Obese Middle-Aged Men with Signs of the Metabolic Syndrome: A Randomised Controlled Trial." *Int J Obes Relat Metab Disord* 25, no. 8 (2001): 1129–35.

Robson V, Dodd S, Thomas S. Standardized antibacterial honey (Medihoney) with standard therapy in wound care: randomized clinical trial. *J Adv Nurs.* 2009 Mar;65(3):565–75.

Rose P, Whiteman M, Moore PK, Zhu YZ. Bioactive S-alk(en)yl cysteine sulfoxide metabolites in the genus Allium: the chemistry of potential therapeutic agents. *Nat Prod Rep.* 2005 Jun;22(3):351–68.

Ruusunen A, Lehto SM, Tolmunen T, Mursu J, Kaplan GA, Voutilainen S. Coffee, tea and caffeine intake and the risk of severe depression in middle-aged Finnish men: the Kuopio Ischaemic Heart Disease Risk Factor Study. *Public Health Nutr.* 2010 Apr 1:1–6.

Sääksjärvi K, Knekt P, Rissanen H, Laaksonen MA, Reunanen A, Männistö S.Prospective study of coffee consumption and risk of Parkinson's disease. *Eur J Clin Nutr.* 2008 Jul;62(7):908–15.

Sanchez-Villegas A, Delgado-Rodriguez M, Alonso A et al. Association of the Mediterranean dietary pattern with the incidence of depression: the Seguimiento Universidad de Navarra/University of Navarra follow-up (SUN) cohort. *Arch Gen Psychiatry.* 2009;66:1090–98.

Sánchez-Villegas A, Verberne L, De Irala J, Ruíz-Canela M, Toledo E, Serra-Majem L, Martínez-González MA. Dietary fat intake and the risk of depression: the SUN Project. *PLoS One.* 2011 Jan 26;6(1):e16268.

Sasaki N, Fukatsu R, Tsuzuki K, Hayashi Y, Yoshida T, Fujii N, Koike T, Wakayama I, Yanagihara R, Garruto R, Amano N, Makita Z. Advanced glycation end products in Alzheimer's disease and other neurodegenerative diseases. *Am J Pathol.* 1998 Oct;153(4):1149–55.

Schab, D. W., and N. H. Trinh. "Do Artificial Food Colors Promote Hyperactivity in Children with Hyperactive Syndromes? A Meta-Analysis of Double-Blind Placebo-Controlled Trials." *J Dev Behav Pediatr* 25, no. 6 (2004): 423-34.

Scrafford CG, Tran NL, Barraj LM, Mink PJ. Egg consumption and CHD and stroke mortality: a prospective study of US adults. *Public Health Nutr.* 2011 Feb;14(2):261–70.

Sen CK, Ann NY. Tocotrienol: the natural vitamin E to defend the nervous system? *Acad Sci.* 2004 Dec;1031:127-42.

Seneff S, Wainwright G, Mascitelli L. Nutrition and Alzheimer's disease: the detrimental role of a high carbohydrate diet. *Eur J Intern Med.* 2011 Apr;22(2):134–40.

Shapiro, A., W. Mu, C. Roncal, K. Y. Cheng, R. J. Johnson, and P. J. Scarpace. "Fructose-Induced Leptin Resistance Exacerbates Weight Gain in Response to Subsequent High-Fat Feeding." *Am J Physiol Regul Integr Comp Physiol* 295, no. 5 (2008): R1370–5.

Shishehbor MH, Brennan ML, Aviles RJ, Fu X, Penn MS, Sprecher DL, Hazen SL. Statins promote potent systemic antioxidant effects through specific inflammatory pathways. *Circulation.* 2003 Jul 29;108(4):426–31.

Simon GE, MD, MPH; Michael Von Korff, ScD; Kathleen Saunders, JD; Diana L. Miglioretti, PhD; Paul K. Crane, MD, MPH; Gerald van Belle, PhD; Ronald C. Kessler, PhD. Association between obesity and psychiatric disorders in the US adult population. *Arch Gen Psychiatry.* 2006;63:824–30.

Slavin JL. Position of the American Dietetic Association: health implications of dietary fiber. *J Am Diet Assoc.* 2008 Oct;108(10):1716–31.

Smith AD, Smith SM, de Jager CA, Whitbread P, Johnston C, Agacinski G, Oulhaj A, Bradley KM, Jacoby R, Refsum H. Homocysteine-lowering by B vitamins slows the rate of accelerated brain atrophy in mild cognitive impairment: a randomized controlled trial. *PLoS One.* 2010 Sep 8;5(9):e12244.

Smith, Andrew. *Eating History: Thirty Turning Points in the Making of American Cuisine.* 2009. Columbia University Press. New York.

Solfrizzi V, Capurso C, D'Introno A, Colacicco AM, Frisardi V, Santamato A, Ranieri M, Fiore P, Vendemiale G, Seripa D, Pilotto A, Capurso A, Panza F. Dietary fatty acids, age-related cognitive decline, and mild cognitive impairment. *J Nutr Health Aging.* 2008 Jun-Jul;12(6):382-6.

Solfrizzi V, Capurso C, D'Introno A, Colacicco AM, Frisardi V, Santamato A, Ranieri M, Fiore P, Vendemiale G, Seripa D, Pilotto A, Capurso A, Panza F. Dietary fatty acids, age-related cognitive decline, and mild cognitive impairment. *J Nutr Health Aging.* 2008 Jun–Jul;12(6):382–86.

Sommerfield AJ, Deary IJ, Frier BM. Acute hyperglycemia alters mood state and impairs cognitive performance in people with type 2 diabetes. *Diabetes Care.* 2004 Oct;27(10):2335–40.

Spangler R, Wittkowski KM, Goddard NL, Avena NM, Hoebel BG, Leibowitz SF. Opiate-like effects of sugar on gene expression in reward areas of the rat brain. *Brain Res Mol Brain Res.* 2004 May 19;124(2):134–42.

Spiller F, Alves MK, Vieira SM, Carvalho TA, Leite CE, Lunardelli A, Poloni JA,

Cunha FQ, de Oliveira JR. Anti-inflammatory effects of red pepper (Capsicum baccatum) on carrageenan- and antigen-induced inflammation. *J Pharm Pharmacol.* 2008 Apr;60(4):473–78.

Stanek KM et al. Obesity is associated with reduced white matter integrity in otherwise healthy adults. *Obesity.* 2011 Mar;19:500. doi:10.1038/oby.2010.312.

Stanhope KL, Havel PJ. Endocrine and metabolic effects of consuming beverages sweetened with fructose, glucose, sucrose, or high-fructose corn syrup. *Am J Clin Nutr.* 2008 Dec;88(6):1733S–37S.

Stanhope KL, Schwarz JM, Keim NL, Griffen SC, Bremer AA, Graham JL, Hatcher B, Cox CL, Dyachenko A, Zhang W, McGahan JP, Seibert A, Krauss RM, Chiu S, Schaefer EJ, Ai M, Otokozawa S, Nakajima K, Nakano T, Beysen C, Hellerstein MK, Berglund L, Havel PJ. Consuming fructose-sweetened, not glucose-sweetened, beverages increases visceral adiposity and lipids and decreases insulin sensitivity in overweight/obese humans. *J Clin Invest.* 2009 May;119(5):1322–34. doi:10.1172/JCI37385.

Sundram K, Karupaiah T, Hayes KC. Stearic acid-rich interesterified fat and trans-rich fat raise the LDL/HDL ratio and plasma glucose relative to palm olein in humans. *Nutr Metab* (Lond). 2007 Jan 15;4:3.

Teff KL, Elliott SS, Tschöp M, Kieffer TJ, Rader D, Heiman M, Townsend RR, Keim NL, D'Alessio D, Havel PJ. Dietary fructose reduces circulating insulin and leptin, attenuates postprandial suppression of ghrelin, and increases triglycerides in women. *J Clin Endocrinol Metab.* 2004 Jun;89(6):2963–72.

Thorve VS, Kshirsagar AD, Vyawahare NS, Joshi VS, Ingale KG, Mohite RJ. Diabetes-induced erectile dysfunction: epidemiology, pathophysiology and management. *J Diabetes Complications.* 2010 May 10.

Todorich B et al. Oligodendrocytes and myelination: the role of iron. *Glia.* 2009 Apr 1;57(5):467–78.

Toverud, Guttorm. A survey of the literature of dental caries. 1952. National Research Council (US) Committee on Dental Health. 422–23.

van Gelder BM, Tijhuis M, Kalmijn S, Kromhout D. Fish consumption, n-3 fatty acids, and subsequent 5-y cognitive decline in elderly men: the Zutphen Elderly Study. *Am J Clin Nutr.* 2007 Apr;85(4):1142–47.

Vincent RP, le Roux CW. The satiety hormone peptide YY as a regulator of appetite. *J Clin Pathol.* 2008 May;61(5):548–52.

Vogiatzoglou A, Refsum H, Johnston C, Smith SM, Bradley KM, de Jager C, Budge MM, Smith AD. Vitamin B12 status and rate of brain volume loss in community-dwelling elderly. *Neurosci Lett.* 1996 Dec 13;220(2):129–32.

Wang SH, Sun ZL, Guo YJ, Yuan Y, Yang BQ. Diabetes impairs hippocampal function via advanced glycation end product mediated new neuron generation in animals with diabetes-related depression. *Toxicol Sci.* 2009 Sep;111(1):72–79.

Wang Y, Ho CT. Polyphenolic chemistry of tea and coffee: a century of progress. *J Agric Food Chem.* 2009 Sep 23;57(18):8109–14.

Wang Y, Jones PJ. Dietary conjugated linoleic acid and body composition. *Am J Clin Nutr.* 2004 Jun;79(6 Suppl):1153S–58S.

Watras AC, Buchholz AC, Close RN, Zhang Z, Schoelle DA. The role of conjugated linoleic acid in reducing body fat and preventing holiday weight gain. *Int J Obes* (Lond). 2007 Mar;31(3), 481–87.

Weese, J. S. "Methicillin-Resistant Staphylococcus Aureus in Animals." *ILAR J* 51, no. 3 (2010): 233–44.

Westover AN, Marangell LB. A cross-national relationship between sugar consumption and major depression? *Depress Anxiety.* 2002;16(3):118–20.

White, L. R., H. Petrovitch, G. W. Ross, K. Masaki, J. Hardman, J. Nelson, D. Davis, and W. Markesbery. "Brain Aging and Midlife Tofu Consumption." *J Am Coll Nutr* 19, no. 2 (2000): 242–55.

Wiles, N. J., K. Northstone, P. Emmett, and G. Lewis. "'Junk Food' Diet and Childhood Behavioural Problems: Results from the Alspac Cohort." *Eur J Clin Nutr* 63, no. 4 (2009): 491–8.

Wilkins CH, Sheline YI, Roe CM, Birge SJ, Morris JC. Vitamin D deficiency is associated with low mood and worse cognitive performance in older adults. *Am J Geriatr Psychiatry.* 2006 Dec;14(12):1032–40.

Wolfe AR, Ogbonna EM, Lim S, Li Y, Zhang J. Dietary linoleic and oleic fatty acids in relation to severe depressed mood: 10 years follow-up of a national cohort. *Prog Neuropsychopharmacol Biol Psychiatry.* 2009 Aug 31;33(6):972–77.

Wong JM, de Souza R, Kendall CW, Emam A, Jenkins DJ. Colonic health: fermentation and short chain fatty acids. *J Clin Gastroenterol.* 2006 Mar;40(3):235–43.

Wurtman RJ, Cansev M, Ulus IH. Synapse formation is enhanced by oral administration of uridine and DHA, the circulating precursors of brain phosphatides. *J Nutr Health Aging.* 2009 Mar;13(3):189–97.

Xia T, Wang Q. Antihyperglycemic effect of Cucurbita ficifolia fruit extract in streptozotocin-induced diabetic rats. *Fitoterapia.* 2006 Dec;77(7–8):530–33.

Yam D, Eliraz A, Berry EM. Diet and disease—the Israeli paradox: possible dangers of a high omega-6 polyunsaturated fatty acid diet. *Isr J Med Sci.* 1996 Nov;32(11):1134–43.

Youdim MB. Brain iron deficiency and excess; cognitive impairment and neurodegeneration with involvement of striatum and hippocampus. *Neurotox Res.* 2008 Aug;14(1):45–56.

Young LR, Nestle M. The contribution of expanding portion sizes to the US obesity epidemic. *Am J Public Health.* 2002 Feb;92(2):246–49.

Zhang R, Humphreys I, Sahu RP, Shi Y, Srivastava SK. In vitro and in vivo induction of apoptosis by capsaicin in pancreatic cancer cells is mediated through ROS generation and mitochondrial death pathway. *Apoptosis.* 2008 Dec;13(12):1465–78.

Zhao N, Zhong C, Wang Y, Zhao Y, Gong N, Zhou G, Xu T, Hong Z. Impaired hippocampal neurogenesis is involved in cognitive dysfunction induced by thiamine deficiency at early pre-pathological lesion stage. *Neurobiol Dis.* 2008 Feb;29(2):176–85.

Index

Underscored page references indicate boxed text.